THE FOOD COMBINING COOKBOOK

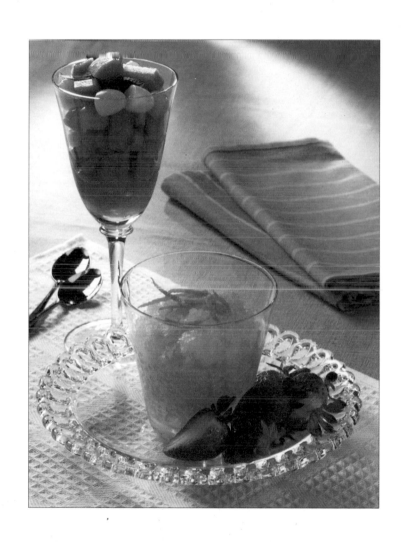

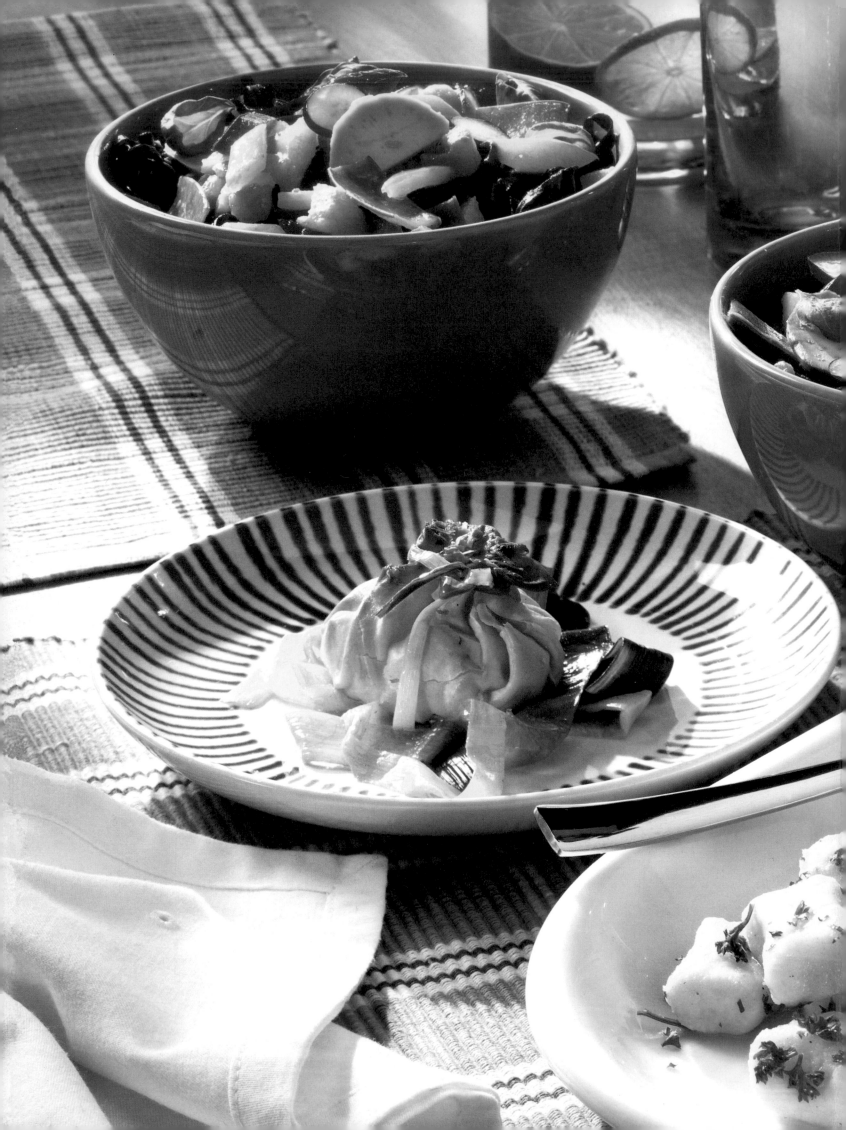

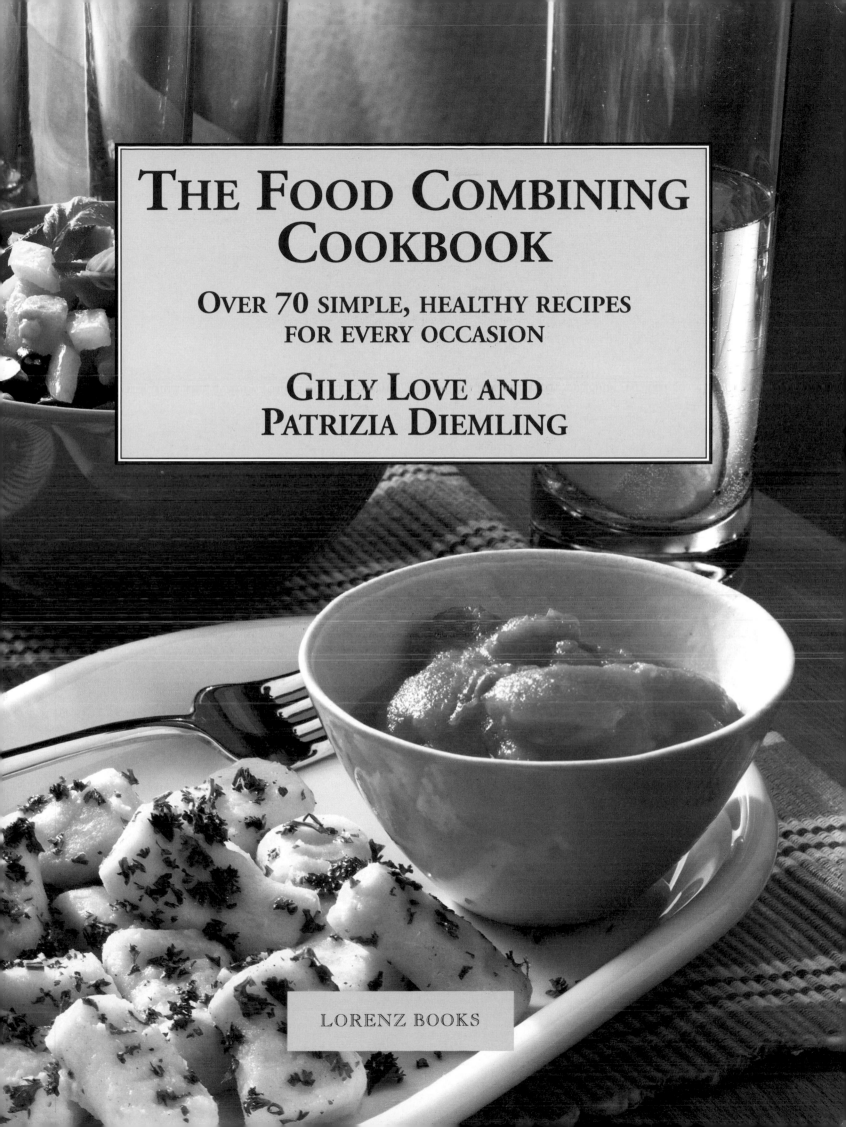

THE FOOD COMBINING COOKBOOK

OVER 70 SIMPLE, HEALTHY RECIPES FOR EVERY OCCASION

GILLY LOVE AND PATRIZIA DIEMLING

LORENZ BOOKS

This edition first published in the USA in 1998 by Lorenz Books
27 West 20th Street, New York, NY 10011

LORENZ BOOKS are available for bulk purchase for sales promotion and for
premium use. For details, write or call the sales director: Anness Publishing Inc.,
27 West 20th Street, New York, NY 10011; (800) 354-9657

Lorenz Books is an imprint of
Anness Publishing Limited

ISBN 1-85967-668-5

Publisher: Joanna Lorenz
Senior Cookbook Editor: Linda Fraser
Copy Editor: Christine Ingram
Indexer: Hilary Bird
Designer: Ian Sandom
Photographer: Thomas Odulate
Food for Photography: Patrizia Diemling, assisted by Mary McCabe
Stylist: Gilly Love
Illustrator: Madeleine David

Printed in Singapore by Star Standard Industries Pte. Ltd.

1 3 5 7 9 10 8 6 4 2

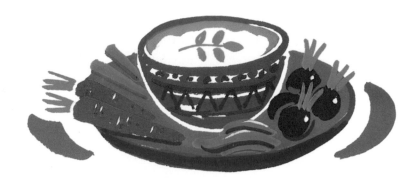

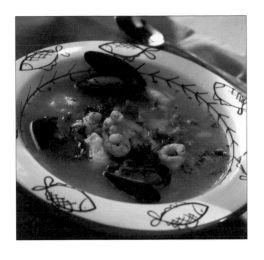
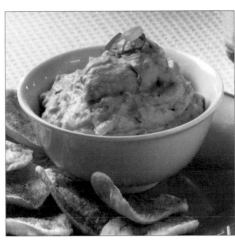
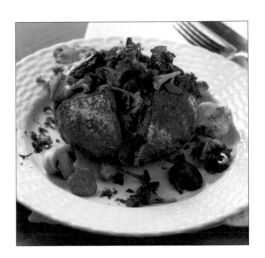

CONTENTS

INTRODUCTION

Some 80 years ago, an American doctor, Dr. William Howard Hay, developed an entirely new system of eating. He had found that a person's health and well-being were largely determined by what they ate. Dr. Hay had suffered from a debilitating kidney disease, but by experimenting with his diet he was able to alleviate the symptoms dramatically.

Over the years since Dr. Hay first developed his theories, thousands of people have found that following the Hay System has improved their health, increased their levels of energy and enabled them to maintain an optimum body weight. Scientific research also points to the fact that a diet that includes plenty of fresh fruit and raw vegetables every day can reduce the chance of developing such conditions as heart disease, strokes and many cancers.

THE HAY SYSTEM

The principles of the Hay system of eating are remarkably simple and they have changed little over the years. Aware that the body contains alkaline and acid mineral salts in a proportion of 4 to 1, Dr. Hay concluded that this balance should be maintained by eating foods with corresponding amounts of alkaline and acid salts. Fruit, most vegetables and herbs are alkaline-forming foods. The Hay system of eating is largely about increasing the consumption of these foods so that our diet mimics the balance in the body.

Hay also found that proteins and carbohydrates, though both acid-forming, need different conditions for digestion and should never be eaten at the same meal. Food combining means using these principles to classify foods and combine compatible foods to provide three basic types of meals—protein, neutral and starch.

FOOD CLASSIFICATION

Food is basically classified as follows:
Alkaline-forming foods: all fresh fruits and green and root vegetables (except starchy vegetables). The Hay diet recommends that we should eat four portions of these foods for every one portion of acid-forming foods. The alkaline- or acid-forming nature of a food has nothing to do with the flavor—some acidic-tasting foods, such as citrus fruits, are good sources of alkaline salts.
Concentrated proteins (acid-forming foods): meat, poultry, game, fish, eggs and cheese.
Concentrated carbohydrates (acid-forming): grains, flours, bread, pasta, rice and all sugars.

Below, clockwise from top: Apples, apricots, passion fruits, dates, oranges, strawberries, raspberries, pears, apricots, blueberries and blackberries, are all alkaline-forming.

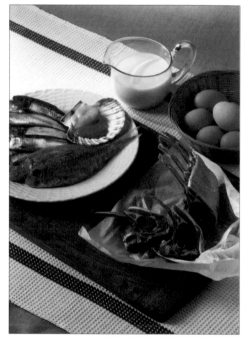

Above: Concentrated protein foods, which are all acid-forming foods, include (clockwise from top) milk, eggs, meat, fish and shellfish, as well as poultry and game.

Dr Hay's Basic Principles
• Never mix concentrated carbohydrates and concentrated proteins. Although both are acid-forming, they are not compatible. Proteins require an acid environment in the digestive tract, while to digest starch most efficiently the body needs an alkaline medium. If the two are mixed, the acid medium is partly neutralized and proteins are then only partly digested.
• Allow 4–5 hours between a starch and a protein meal.
• Make fresh fruits and vegetables form the major part of your daily eating. Try to eat three or four portions of fruit, vegetables or salad every day. Ideally they should be raw, or in the case of vegetables, lightly steamed or stir-fried.

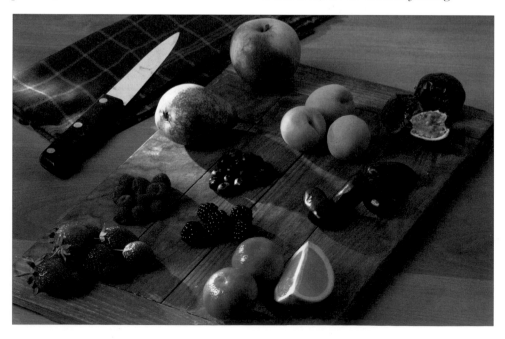

• Avoid all processed and refined foods. This is another important rule, although quite hard to follow, as so much of our food—canned beans, cookies, cakes, frozen dinners and so on—comes in processed form. Get into the habit of making your own homemade cakes and cookies and, whenever possible, use whole grains rather than the refined white alternative, be it pasta, rice, bread or flour.

The following table gives a quick reference as to which foods are compatible. It divides foods into three separate food groups: protein, neutral and starch. The neutral foods may be combined with *either* protein foods *or* starch foods. The important rule is *never* to mix protein foods and starch foods in the same meal.

Protein Foods	Neutral Foods	Starch Foods
Meat	Butter	Cereals—wheat, barley, rye, millet, cornmeal and oats
Poultry	Cream and crème fraîche	
Game	Cream cheese	Bread
Fish and shellfish	Egg yolks	Flour
Whole eggs	Olive oil, sunflower oil, sesame oil and walnut oil	Oatmeal
Cheese		Very sweet fruits—bananas, very ripe pears, papaya, very sweet grapes, figs, dates and dried fruits
Milk and yogurt★	All nuts, except peanuts	
	Nut and seed butters, except peanut butter	
All fruits except very sweet fruits (*see* Starch Foods)	All green and root vegetables, except starchy vegetables (*see* Starch Foods)	Legumes and beans, except soy beans
Soy beans and tofu		Peanuts and peanut butter
Cooked tomatoes	All salads and sprouted beans and seeds	Starchy vegetables—potatoes, yams, sweet potatoes, corn and Jerusalem artichokes
Lemon tea		
Grape juice, the less sweet varieties	All herbs and spices	Sweet grape juice
	Honey and maple syrup	
Tomato juice, canned and vacuum-packed	Water	Beer, ale and stout
		Sweet wines and liqueurs
Dry wines and dry cider	Herb teas	
	Tomato juice, fresh	
★Milk and yogurt are classified as protein foods, but a little of either can be combined with starch	All vegetable juices	
	Yeast-extract drinks	
	Gin and most liquors	
	Weak coffee or tea in moderation	

Note that this table should be used for checking the compatibility of foods. It is not concerned with whether foods are alkaline- or acid-forming.

CAN I DO IT?

Although at first glance, a food combining diet seems complicated and prescriptive, you will find in a surprisingly short time how easy and enjoyable it is. It is important not to think in terms of "giving up" all those mixed meals, such as cheese sandwiches and fish fry suppers. Instead, concentrate on the positive side. Sandwiches made with whole-wheat bread or pitas and stuffed with salad can be equally delicious. Or try Roasted Cod with Fresh Tomato Sauce served with a generous portion of Baked Vegetable Chips. Many people who follow this system of eating are delighted to find that they gradually lose excess pounds, without ever once feeling hungry. In addition, all the meals contained in this book are suitable for family eating, so if your principal intention for following the system is to lose weight, you will not feel isolated, but can continue enjoying meals with family and friends. The recipes in this book are simple and relatively quick to prepare and cook. As well as many tasty suggestions for family eating, there are also recipes for more sophisticated meals, from luncheons to dinner parties. The occasional treat is included, and there are delicious desserts to combine with both protein and starch main courses, as well as a choice of homemade breads and cakes.

USING THIS BOOK

Each recipe is labeled individually with a "P" to indicate a protein dish or an "S" to show a starch dish. "N" means the dish is neutral, which indicates it can be combined with either a protein or a starch meal. If, for instance, you want to serve Lentil Risotto with Vegetables (S), you can first serve Gazpacho Salsa (N). This salsa also can be served with Salmon with Yogurt and Mint Dressing (P). Try to balance your daily menu, so that you have one starch, one protein and one neutral dish a day.

INGREDIENTS

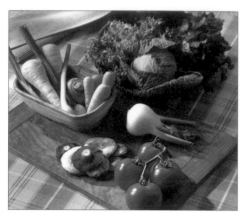

Above: Vegetables that are neutral include (clockwise from top): lettuce, cabbage, fennel, tomatoes, mushrooms, carrots, turnips, parsnips and scallions.

FRUITS

It would be difficult to overstate the importance of fresh fruit in a healthy diet. Recent studies in the U.S. and England have testified to its protective role as regards health. Try to eat at least two pieces of preferably raw fruit each day. Ideally, it should be eaten on an empty stomach, since the digestion of fruit is much faster when it is eaten on its own. Alternatively, leave 15 minutes between courses, so that fruit can digest partly by itself. This is particularly important with melon, which does not digest well with other food.

Fruit is an excellent way to start the day, as the natural sugars provide instant energy. Most fruits can precede or follow a protein course. For starch meals, choose very sweet fruits, such as ripe bananas, papayas or pears. Dried fruits—such as dates, raisins and figs—are also better combined with starch meals.

Always be sure to choose fruit in peak condition and, if possible, buy the organic variety. Lemons, especially if you are using the rind for flavoring or dressing, should be unwaxed.

VEGETABLES AND SALADS

Vegetables and salads are also enormously important in a food combining diet. All green and root vegetables, together with salads and herbs, are deemed neutral, which means they can be combined with either protein or starch foods. The exceptions are vegetables such as potatoes, sweet potatoes, Jerusalem artichokes, corn and yams, which have high starch content and are not compatible with protein meals. Tomatoes, on the other hand, though neutral when raw, become very acidic once cooked and should be combined only with protein dishes.

Always make sure vegetables are absolutely fresh and preferably organic. Although these are likely to cost a little more, vegetables are so central to a food combining diet that you will find it worth spending extra in this area, since you will need to buy less in the way of meat, poultry and fish. Vegetables will become the centerpiece of a meal, while proteins and carbohydrates, though still important in dietary terms, will be featured less, becoming almost the accompaniment to the star attraction—vegetables and salads.

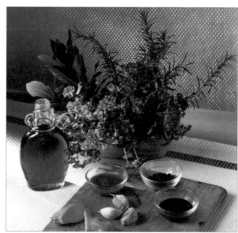

Above: Neutral foods include (clockwise from top) fresh herbs, peppercorns, yeast extract, garlic, fresh ginger, maple syrup and chili sauce.

HERBS AND SPICES

Fresh herbs are indispensable ingredients in a food combining diet. Being neutral, like vegetables, they can be used with either protein or starch meals, where they not only add their own flavor but bring intrinsic nutritional benefit too. Many, like mint and bay, aid digestion, while parsley and chervil are rich in Vitamins A and C. Use fresh herbs whenever possible, for flavor and nutritional value. Many herbs can be grown in the garden or in pots on the kitchen windowsill and this is the best way to ensure that you have a constant and always fresh supply.

Similarly, spices also should be as fresh as possible, so buy small quantities of the whole seeds and grind in a coffee grinder or spice mill. Black pepper should be freshly ground to ensure freshness and always use sea salt, preferably grinding this too in a salt mill.

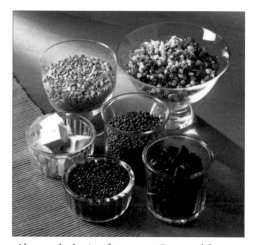

Above, clockwise from top: Sprouted beans, kidney beans, lentils, tofu, sunflower seeds and mung beans (center) are all good sources of protein.

PROTEIN FOODS

Protein is essential in a healthy diet but we need only small quantities. Meat and fish, together with eggs and dairy products, are the best sources of protein. If possible, buy organic meat and free-range chicken. Eggs should always be free-range. Grains, beans and nuts are also good sources of protein and should be a regular part of a vegetarian diet. Sprouted seeds and beans contain living enzymes that help promote good digestion, tissue growth and repair. Unlike many dried beans, which are frequently hard to digest, sprouted seeds and beans are easily digested and are compatible with both protein and starch meals.

SWEETENERS

Refined sugar should be avoided as much as possible. Honey, maple syrup or sweet fruits such as dates, figs and raisins can be used to sweeten desserts.

SPROUTING BEANS, SEEDS AND LEGUMES

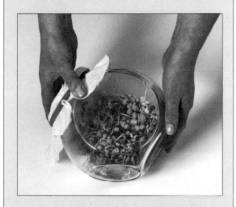

Green and brown lentils; dried mung, aduki, haricot, flageolet and soy beans; whole dried peas, chickpeas and seeds, such as sunflower and pumpkin, will sprout successfully. Ready-made sprouters are available at health food stores. If there is no visible sign of germination after about 48 hours, the beans are probably old and will never grow.

To sprout beans, seeds and legumes, place 3 tablespoons beans, seeds or legumes in a large, wide-mouthed jar and cover with 1 cup fresh tepid water. Cover the jar with muslin, secure with a rubber band and let sit overnight. Remove the cover and rinse the beans thoroughly with fresh tepid water. Drain well, replace the cover and turn the jar on its side, spacing out the beans, seeds or legumes. Keep the jar in a warm room, out of direct sunlight. Rinse the beans, seeds or legumes daily through the muslin top. The sprouts are ready to eat when there is about ½ inch of shoot showing. Rinse and drain thoroughly, then store for up to 2 days in a plastic bag in the refrigerator.

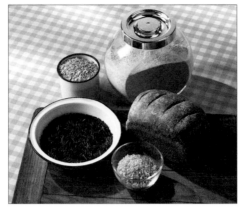

Above: Whole grain foods, such as whole-wheat flour and bread, brown rice, wild rice and oats, are concentrated carbohydrates.

STARCH FOODS

Starches are concentrated carbohydrates; they are an essential part of our diet, providing energy for the body. The best starches are found in whole grains. Choose whole-wheat bread, flour and pasta, and brown rice as opposed to white. For special occasions, a little white flour does no harm, providing your diet contains plenty of the fiber found in fruit and vegetables.

FATS AND OILS

All fats and oils, including butter, egg yolks, olive oil, sunflower oil, cream cheese, cream and crème fraîche, are neutral foods and can be combined with either protein or starch meals. Avoid margarines and low-fat spreads, as they are highly processed.

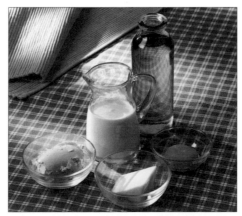

Above, clockwise from top: Olive oil, egg yolk, butter, cream cheese and cream are neutral foods.

Some fat is essential in a healthy diet, but most experts agree that we eat far more than is required. A food combining diet is generally low in fat, partly because it eliminates the hidden fats found in cookies and cakes.

FRESH STOCKS

Fish and vegetable stock are used extensively in the recipes in this book, and while there are some excellent stock cubes and vegetable bouillon powders available, nothing quite matches the flavor of homemade stock. Both can be frozen successfully, but are best if freshly made.

FISH STOCK (P)

To make about 5 cups fish stock, thoroughly wash 1½ pounds white fish bones and trimmings. Melt 1 tablespoon butter in a large, heavy saucepan and fry 1 ounce chopped onion, 2–3 chopped leeks (white part only) and ½ cup chopped mushrooms. Add the fish trimmings, 1 fresh dill sprig, 5 cups water and ½ cup dry white wine. Bring to a boil, then simmer for 20 minutes, occasionally skimming the surface to remove any fat. Strain through a fine sieve.

FRESH VEGETABLE STOCK (N)

To make about 4 cups vegetable stock, chop 4 carrots, 4 stalks celery, 1 large onion, 1 leek and ½ fennel bulb into small dice. Melt 2 tablespoons unsalted butter in a large, heavy saucepan and fry the vegetables together with 1 fresh bay leaf, 1 fresh thyme sprig, 1 small bunch parsley, 1 crushed garlic clove, 5 black peppercorns and a pinch of sea salt over low heat for about 8 minutes, stirring occasionally. Add 5 cups water and simmer for 30 minutes. Pour the stock through a sieve, squeezing out all the vegetable juices with the back of a wooden spoon.

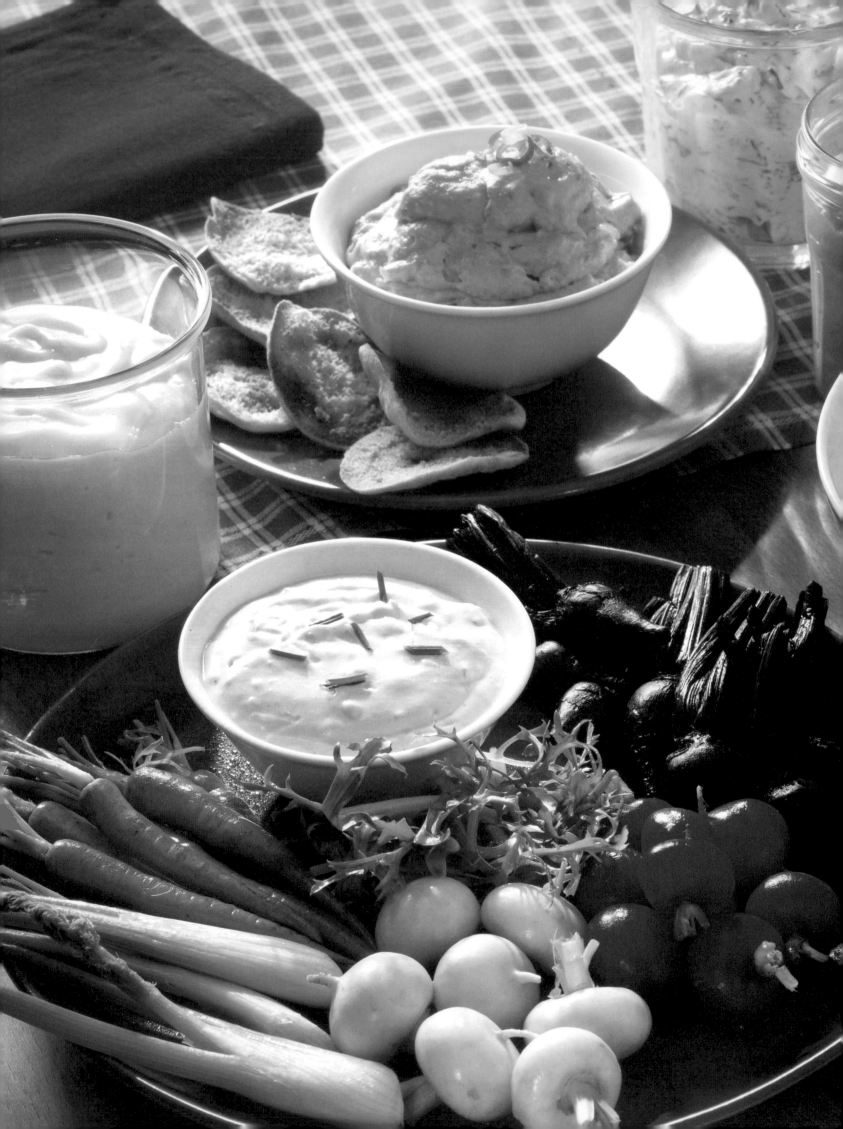

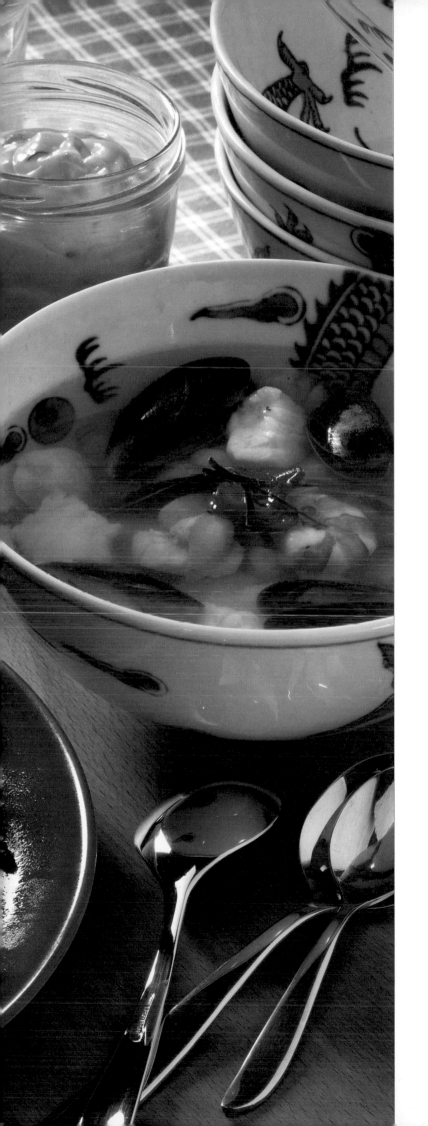

APPETIZERS AND SOUPS

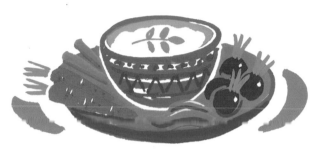

A colorful selection of raw vegetables and salad greens is the most satisfying and healthy way to start each meal. Choose only the freshest seasonal varieties, prepared and served immediately for the best flavor. Serve with Tahini Tofu Dressing followed by a protein main course or Sour Cream and Avocado Dipping Sauce with any starch dish. Warming Italian Arugula and Potato Soup is ideal for winter lunches or as a nutritious supper. And, if you double the portions for Thai Fish Soup, it makes a fragrantly flavored protein main course.

Sour Cream and Avocado Dipping Sauce (N)

Serve with Vegetable Salad (see below) as a neutral appetizer before any main course, or with crisp rounds of toasted pita bread before a starch main course.

INGREDIENTS

Serves 4
1 large ripe avocado
10 fresh chives
juice of 1 lime
1 tablespoon fresh cilantro
1 tablespoon finely chopped scallion
3 tablespoons sour cream
salt and freshly ground black pepper
shreds of scallions, to garnish

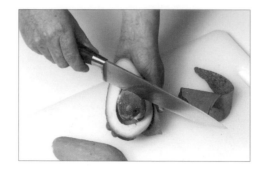

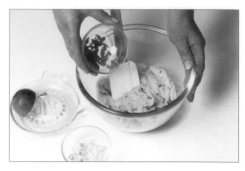

1 Place the avocado in a pan of boiling water and turn continuously for one minute. Remove from the pan and peel away the skin— it should come off easily. Cut the avocado in half and remove the pit.

2 Mash the avocado in a bowl with a fork until the flesh is completely smooth, then snip in the fresh chives.

3 Stir in the lime juice, cilantro and scallion and mix well, then fold in the sour cream and seasoning. Chill for 1 hour before serving, garnished with scallion shreds.

Vegetable Salad (N) with Tahini Tofu Dressing (P)

Choose fresh raw vegetables and salad greens that are in season and, if possible, buy organic varieties (or better still, grow your own). Serve this neutral salad and protein dressing before any neutral or protein main course.

INGREDIENTS

Serves 4
1¼ pounds mixed young raw
  vegetables, washed

For the dressing
1 garlic clove
¼ cup tahini
½ package (4 ounces) soft silken tofu
2 tablespoons lemon juice
¼ cup sunflower oil
1 scallion, finely chopped
1 tablespoon light soy sauce
about ¼ cup water
½ teaspoon finely ground salt

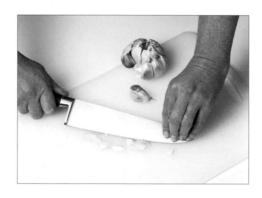

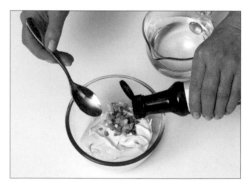

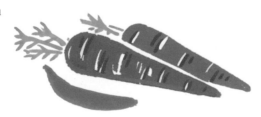

1 Crush the garlic with the blade of a knife, place it in a small bowl and stir in the tahini. Stir in the tofu and lemon juice and then slowly drizzle in the oil.

2 Add the scallion, reserving a few of the green ends as a garnish. Add the soy sauce and stir in enough water to make a smooth, thick cream. Season with salt and spoon into a bowl. Garnish with the reserved scallion and serve with the prepared vegetables.

> ——— COOK'S TIP ———
>
> This dressing can be made in a blender or food processor if desired. Store in an airtight jar in the refrigerator for up to a week.

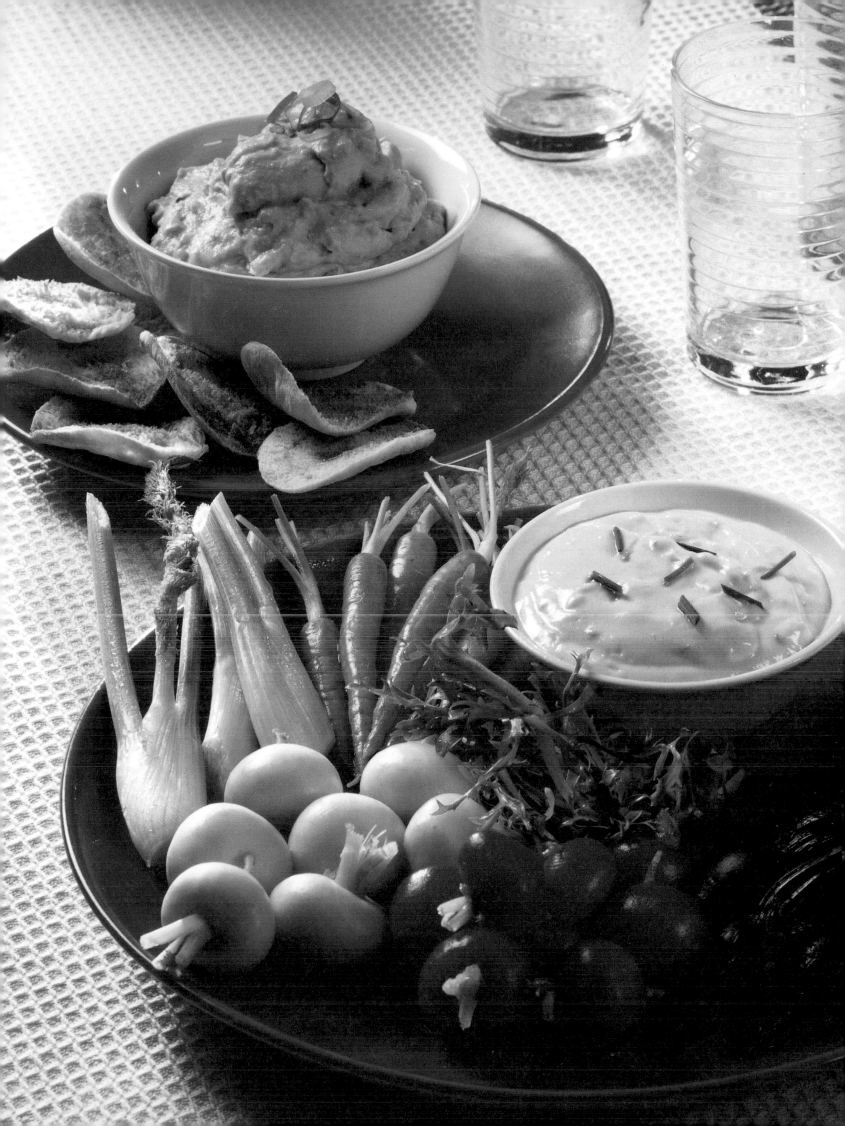

Fresh Cilantro and Yogurt Dipping Sauce (P)

Cilantro is a widely used herb featured in Indian, Mexican, Chinese, Indonesian, Middle Eastern and Caribbean cooking. It is generally available in supermarkets.

INGREDIENTS

Serves 4
1 small bunch fresh cilantro
1 garlic clove
1 small shallot, chopped finely
½ cup plain yogurt
salt and freshly ground black pepper
fresh cilantro sprig, to garnish
    (optional)

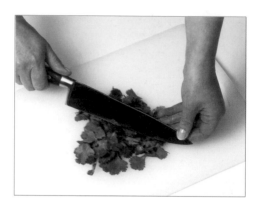

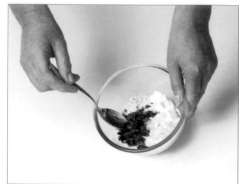

1 Chop the cilantro using a very sharp knife.

2 Using the flat side of a knife blade, crush the garlic with a little salt to absorb the flavor.

3 Mix the cilantro, garlic, shallot and yogurt in a bowl and season to taste with salt and pepper.

4 Spoon into a small serving dish or jar. Serve garnished with a sprig of cilantro, if desired.

Right, clockwise from top left: Fresh Cilantro and Yogurt Dipping Sauce, Saffron-flavored Mayonnaise, Fresh Mayonnaise and Herb-flavored Mayonnaise.

COOK'S TIP

This sauce will keep for 48 hours if stored in a covered container in the refrigerator.

Fresh Mayonnaise (N)

Fresh mayonnaise is a wonderful, versatile dressing. Since it is a neutral food, it can be used for both starch and protein salads.

INGREDIENTS

Serves 4
2 large egg yolks (preferably
    free-range)
½ teaspoon salt
1 teaspoon Dijon mustard
1 teaspoon finely grated lemon rind
    (preferably from an unwaxed lemon)
⅔ cup sunflower oil

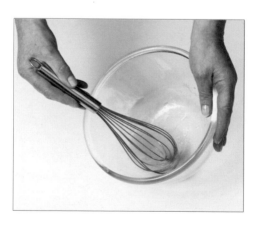

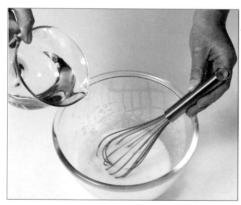

1 Whisk the egg yolks together with the salt, mustard and lemon rind.

2 Add the oil in a slow drizzle, whisking continuously. Do this very slowly at first, so that each drop of oil is incorporated. As the mayonnaise begins to thicken, add the oil in a slow and steady stream. Adjust the seasoning, then spoon the mayonnaise into a serving dish or jar. Mayonnaise can be kept in the refrigerator for 3–4 days. Serve at room temperature.

VARIATIONS

Add finely chopped mixed fresh herbs, or ½ teaspoon saffron threads that have been soaked in 1 tablespoon water.

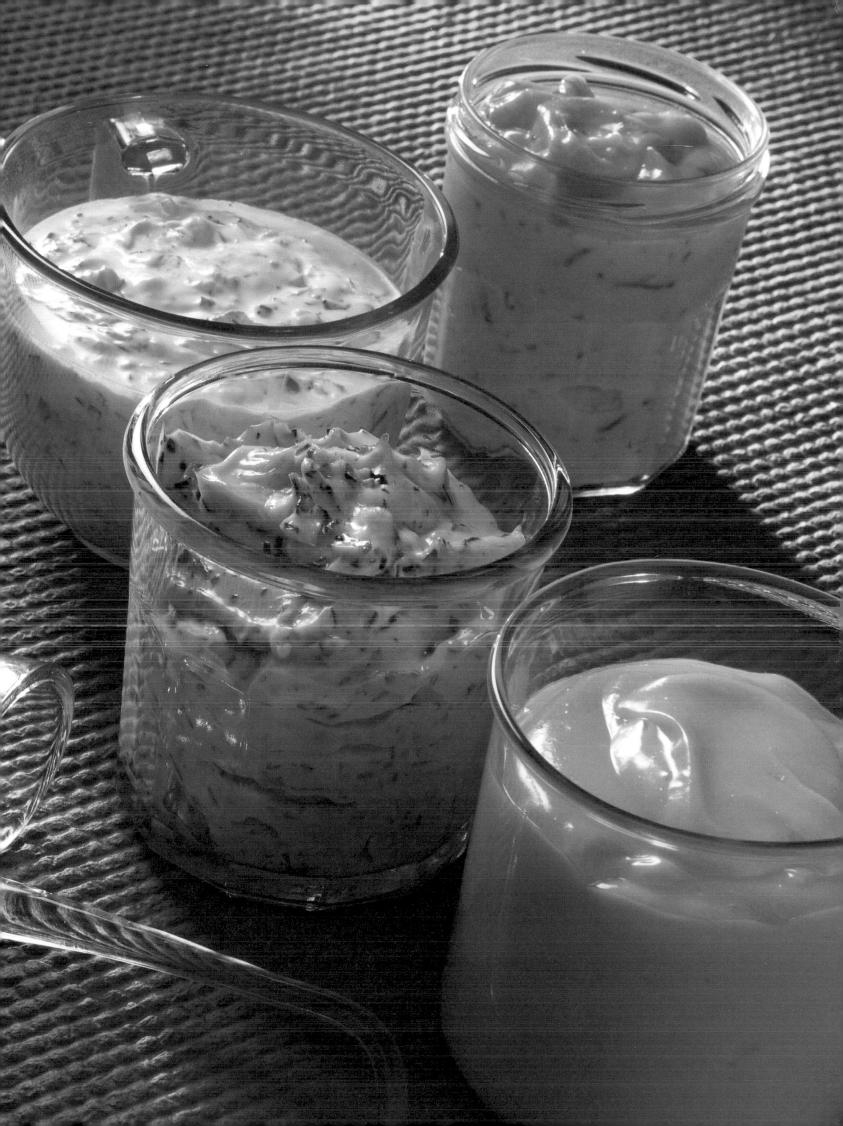

Gazpacho Salsa (N)

Freshly made salsa is delicious with simply grilled or broiled fish. If you can, use homegrown tomatoes for the best flavor. Failing this, pay a little extra for organic tomatoes or buy one of the super-sweet varieties.

INGREDIENTS

Serves 4

½ large or 1 small cucumber
1 small red onion
1 pound firm tomatoes, peeled and seeded
1 large yellow bell pepper
2 fresh red chilies
1 garlic clove, finely chopped
1 tablespoon finely chopped fresh flat-leaf parsley
2 tablespoons finely chopped fresh cilantro
2 tablespoons extra virgin olive oil
1 tablespoon cider vinegar
salt and freshly ground black pepper

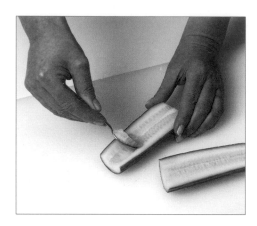

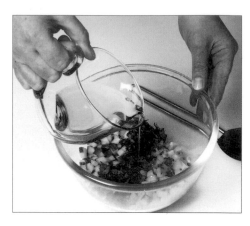

1 Cut the cucumber in half lengthwise. Using a teaspoon, remove and discard the seeds and then cut the flesh into small cubes.

2 Chop the onion and tomatoes into small pieces. Quarter the pepper, discard the seeds and core and cut into small cubes.

3 Finely chop the chilies, discarding the seeds and core.

4 Place all the vegetables in a large bowl and add the garlic, herbs, olive oil, vinegar and seasoning. Combine thoroughly and then chill in the refrigerator for 1 hour. Strain off any excess juices and serve.

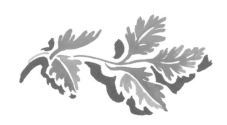

Anchovy and Parsley Relish (P)

Anchovies and parsley make a flavorful relish to serve as a topping for fresh vegetables.

INGREDIENTS

Serves 4

1 small bunch flat-leaf parsley
½ cup black olives, pitted
¼ cup sun-dried tomatoes
4 canned anchovy fillets, drained
½ cup finely chopped red onion
1 tablespoon pickled capers, rinsed
1 garlic clove, finely chopped
1 tablespoon olive oil
juice of ½ lime
¼ teaspoon ground black pepper
a selection of cherry tomatoes, celery and cucumber, to serve

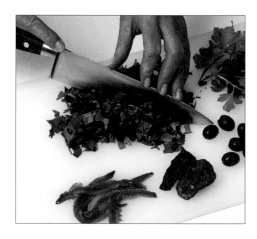

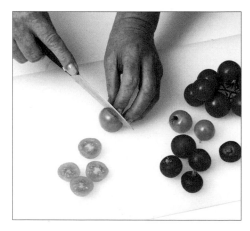

1 Coarsely chop the parsley, black olives, sun-dried tomatoes and anchovy fillets and mix in a bowl with the onion, capers, garlic, olive oil, lime juice and black pepper.

2 Halve the cherry tomatoes, cut the celery into bite-size chunks and cut the cucumber into ½-inch slices. Top each of the prepared vegetables with a generous amount of relish and serve.

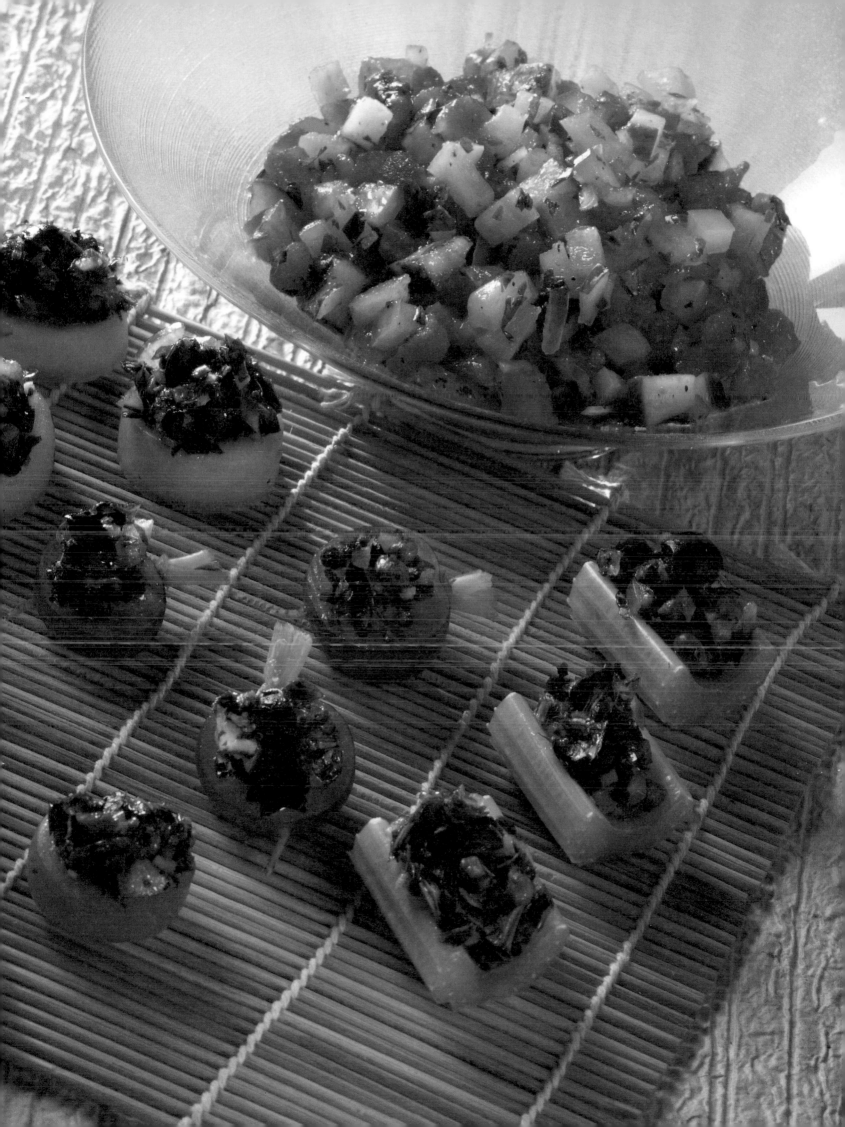

Arugula and Potato Soup (S)

This hearty soup is based on a traditional Italian peasant recipe. If arugula is unavailable, watercress or baby spinach leaves make an equally delicious alternative.

INGREDIENTS

Serves 4

2 pounds new potatoes
4 cups well-seasoned vegetable stock
1 medium carrot
1 bunch arugula
½ teaspoon cayenne pepper
½ loaf stale ciabatta bread, torn into chunks
4 garlic cloves, thinly sliced
¼ cup olive oil
salt and freshly ground black pepper

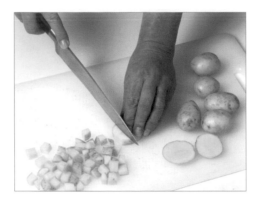

1 Dice the potatoes, then place them in a saucepan with the stock and a little salt. Bring to a boil and simmer for 10 minutes.

--- COOK'S TIP ---

Garlic burns very easily, so keep an eye on the pan!

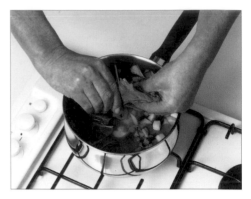

2 Finely dice the carrot and add to the potatoes and stock, then tear the arugula leaves and drop into the pan. Simmer for another 15 minutes, until the vegetables are tender.

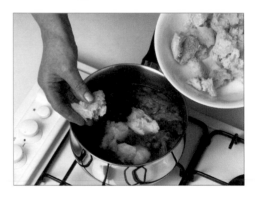

3 Add the cayenne pepper and seasoning, then add the chunks of bread. Remove the pan from the heat, then cover and let stand for about 10 minutes.

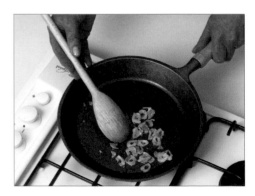

4 Meanwhile, sauté the garlic in the olive oil until golden brown. Pour the soup into bowls, add a little of the sautéed garlic to each bowl and serve.

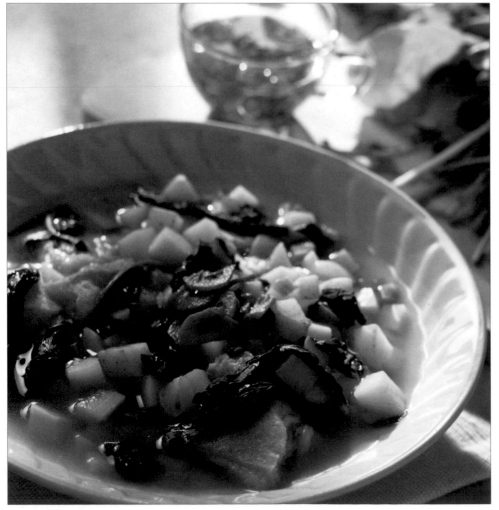

Cream of Roasted Bell Pepper Soup (N)

Weight for weight, red and yellow bell peppers have four times as much Vitamin C as oranges. This is a light, creamy and nutritious soup. Serve with Vegetable Chips instead of Melba toast before a fish main course.

INGREDIENTS

Serves 4
3 large red bell peppers, halved and seeded
1 large yellow bell pepper, halved and seeded
1 tablespoon olive oil
1 small shallot, chopped
2½ cups vegetable stock
2 garlic cloves, crushed
¼ teaspoon saffron strands
½ cup light cream
2 cups water
salt and freshly ground black pepper
sprigs of fresh chervil or flat-leaf parsley, to garnish

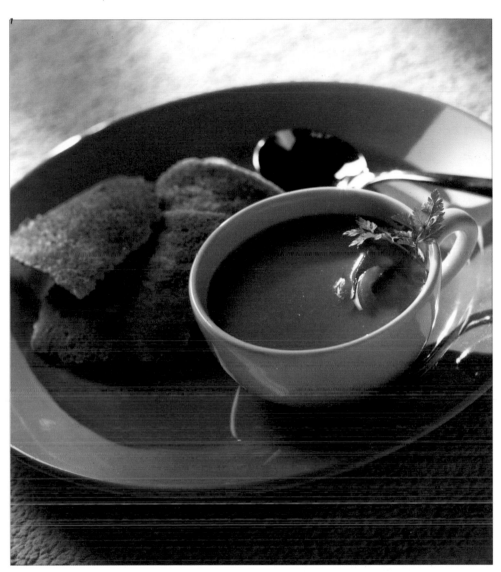

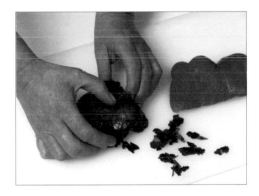

1 Arrange the peppers skin side up on a baking tray and place under a very hot broiler. Broil the peppers until the skin is blackened and blistered, then place them in a plastic bag, knot the end and let sit until cool enough to handle. Peel off the skins, reserve one quarter each of a red and yellow pepper and chop the remaining peppers into rough pieces.

2 Heat the oil in a heavy saucepan and sauté the shallot until transparent and soft. Add the vegetable stock, garlic, saffron and chopped peppers. Bring to a boil and simmer for 15 minutes.

3 Cool for 10 minutes, then process in a blender or food processor until smooth.

COOK'S TIP

If possible, use homemade vegetable stock, or stock made from a good-quality bouillon cube or bouillon powder.

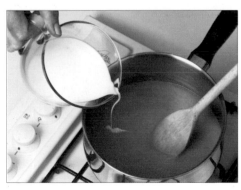

4 Return the soup to a clean pan. Mix together the cream and water and add to the pan with salt and pepper to taste. Reheat gently without boiling. Pour the soup into warmed bowls and garnish with thin strips of the reserved peppers and sprigs of chervil. Serve with Melba toast.

Thai Fish Soup (P)

Nam pla is a Thai fish sauce, rich in B vitamins, that is used extensively in Thai cooking. It is available at Thai or Indonesian stores and good supermarkets.

INGREDIENTS

Serves 4

8 jumbo shrimp
1 lime
1 tablespoon peanut oil
5 cups well-seasoned chicken or fish stock
1 lemongrass stalk, bruised, cut into 1-inch lengths
2 kaffir lime leaves, torn into pieces
½ fresh green chili, seeded and finely sliced
4 large scallops
24 mussels, scrubbed
4 ounces monkfish fillet, cut into ¾-inch chunks
1 tablespoon *nam pla*
1 kaffir lime leaf, ½ red chili, ½ lemongrass stalk, sliced, to garnish

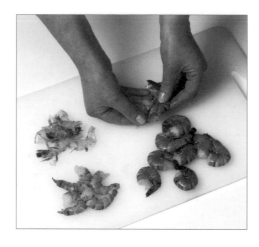

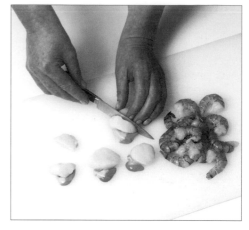

1 Peel the shrimp, reserving the shells, and remove the black thread along the back. Grate the lime rind and squeeze the juice.

2 Heat the oil in a saucepan and fry the shrimp shells until pink. Add the chicken stock, lemongrass, kaffir lime leaves, lime rind and sliced green chili. Bring to a boil, simmer for 20 minutes and then strain through a fine sieve, reserving the liquid.

3 Prepare the scallops by cutting them in half, leaving the corals (if any) attached to one half.

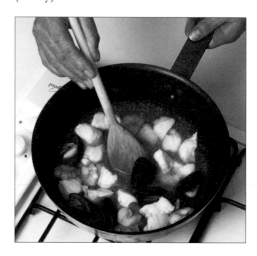

4 Return the stock to a clean pan, add the shrimp, mussels, monkfish and scallops and cook for 3 minutes. Remove from the heat and add the lime juice and *nam pla*.

5 Serve garnished with finely sliced red chili, lemongrass and the kaffir lime leaf.

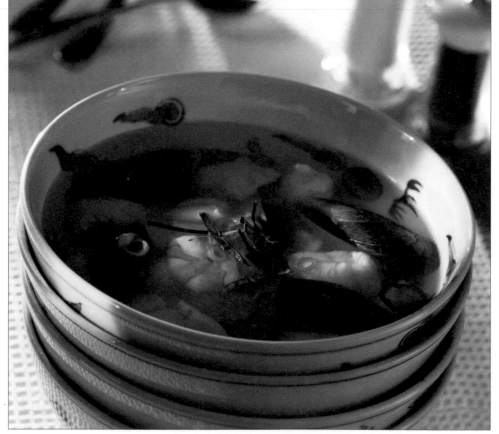

COOK'S TIP

Double the quantity of fish and seafood to serve as a protein main course.

Stargazer Vegetable Soup (S)

If you have the time, it is worth making your own stock for this recipe—either vegetable or, if you prefer, chicken or fish.

INGREDIENTS

Serves 4
1 yellow bell pepper
2 large zucchini
2 large carrots
1 kohlrabi
4 cups well-seasoned vegetable stock
2 ounces rice vermicelli
salt and freshly ground black pepper

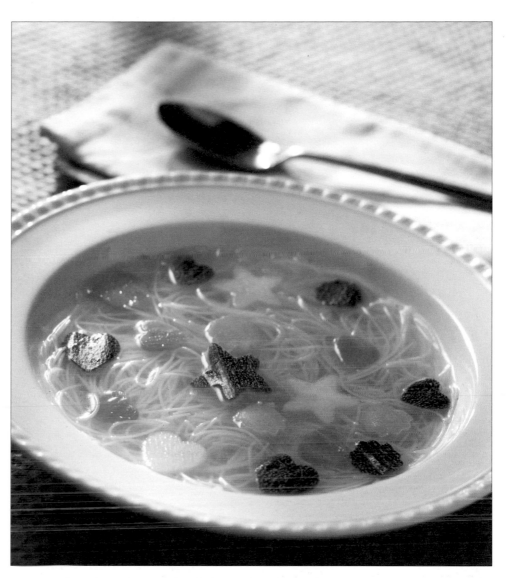

1 Cut the pepper into quarters, removing the seeds and core. Cut the zucchini and carrots lengthwise into ¼-inch slices and slice the kohlrabi into ¼-inch rounds.

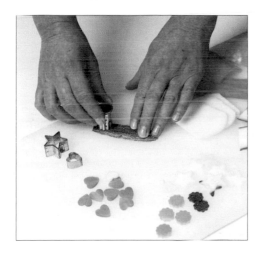

2 Using tiny cookie cutters, stamp out star shapes from the vegetables or use a very sharp knife to fashion the sliced vegetables into stars and other decorative shapes.

COOK'S TIP

Sauté the remaining vegetable pieces in a little oil and mix with cooked brown rice to make a tasty risotto.

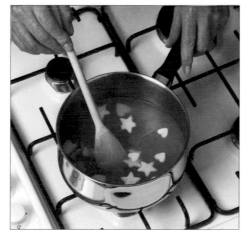

3 Place the vegetables and stock in a pan and simmer for 10 minutes. Season to taste with salt and pepper.

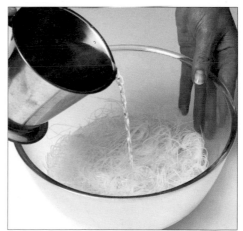

4 Meanwhile, place the vermicelli in a bowl, cover with boiling water and set aside for 4 minutes. Drain, divide among four warmed soup bowls and ladle in the soup.

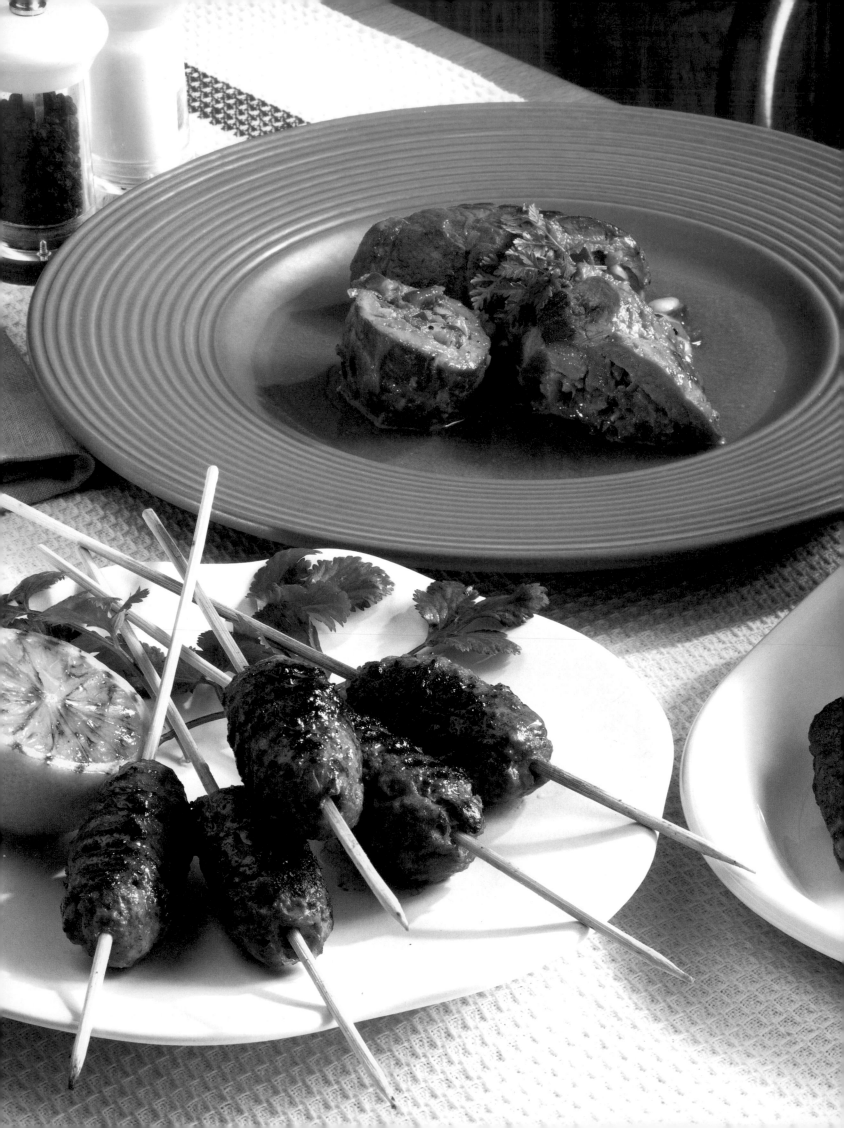

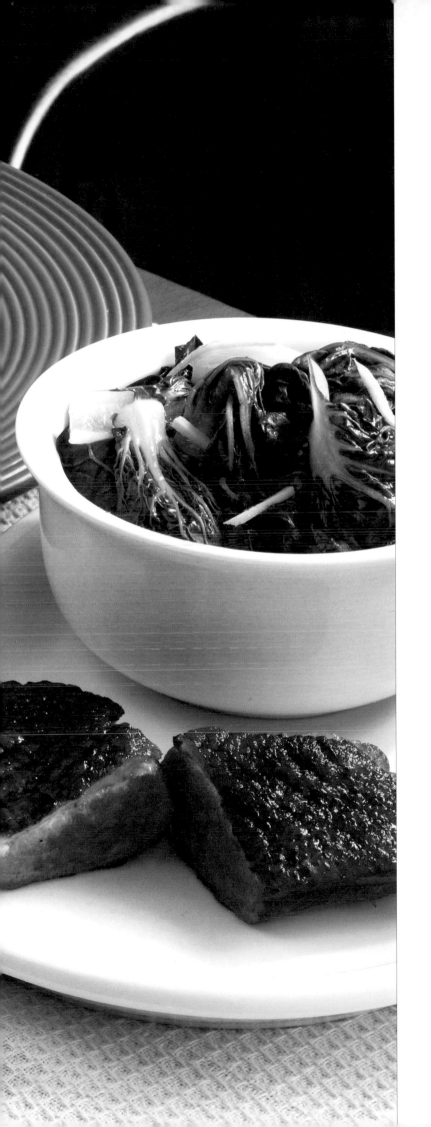

MEAT AND POULTRY

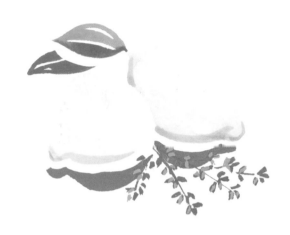

You don't have to be a vegetarian to enjoy a healthy diet. If you do buy meat, choose lean, fresh and preferably organic meats or poultry and game with the skin removed. Free-range chicken has a delicate flavor and, when lightly poached in an aromatic broth, makes a delightful summer lunch, served with a sharp, mustardy mayonnaise. Chicken is delicious with Thai-inspired creamy coconut sauce or stir-fried with Chinese sauces, fresh ginger and lime. For special occasions, entertain your guests with pheasant breasts gently flavored with caramelized apples or crispy duck breasts and bok choy.

Pork Fillet with Bell Pepper and Pine Nuts (P)

Pork fillet, also known as tenderloin, is a very lean and inexpensive cut of meat. The tasty stuffing not only adds flavor, but also keeps the meat moist during cooking. Serve with vegetable purée and lots of lightly steamed broccoli.

INGREDIENTS

Serves 4

¼ cup peanut oil
2 shallots, finely chopped
4 garlic cloves, finely chopped
2 red bell peppers, seeded and cut into
    small pieces
½ cup pine nuts
1 tablespoon chopped fresh chervil
2 pork fillets, about 12 ounces each
1¼ cups medium-dry white wine
1¼ cups chicken stock
1 teaspoon saffron threads
salt and freshly ground black pepper
sprigs of fresh chervil, to garnish

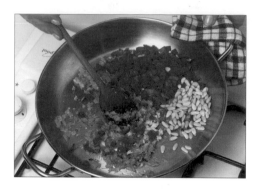

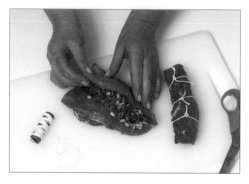

1 Preheat the oven to 375°F. Heat 2 tablespoons of the oil in a large heavy ovenproof frying pan. Add the shallots and fry gently for 4 minutes, until soft, then stir in the garlic, peppers and pine nuts and sauté for another 5 minutes, stirring occasionally. Remove from the heat and add the chervil and seasoning.

2 Split each pork fillet lengthwise without cutting right through and open up each one like a book. Place the pork fillets between two sheets of plastic wrap and lightly flatten with a rolling pin.

3 Spoon the pepper mixture down the center of each pork fillet. Fold the meat carefully over the filling and secure with cotton string tied at 1-inch intervals.

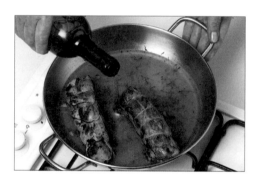

4 Heat the remaining oil in the frying pan and fry the fillets for a few minutes, until evenly brown. Add the wine, stock and saffron, then cover and bake for about 25 minutes or until the meat is cooked through. Remove the lid or foil and cook, uncovered, for another 10 minutes to brown.

5 Transfer the pork fillets to a serving plate and keep warm. Pour the cooking liquid into a saucepan, bring to a boil and cook until reduced by half. Season to taste and pour into a serving pitcher.

6 Slice the meat thickly, remembering to remove the string, and serve with the sauce, garnished with sprigs of fresh chervil.

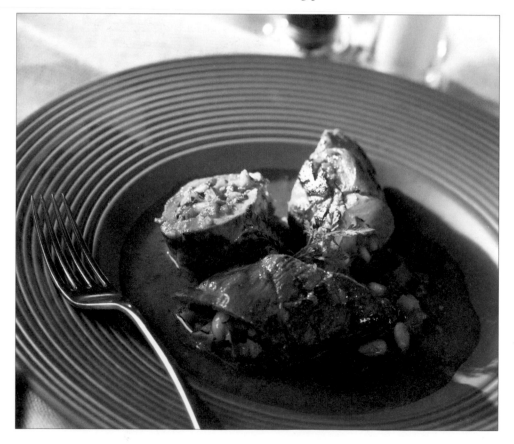

Pheasant Breasts with Caramelized Apples (P)

Game is free-range meat that is naturally low in saturated fat. By cooking these pheasant breasts quickly and gently, you retain all their tenderness and flavor. Use free-range chicken breasts when pheasant is unavailable or for a more economical meal.

INGREDIENTS

Serves 4

4 pheasant breasts, about 6 ounces
    each, skinned
4 tablespoons (½ stick) unsalted butter
1 teaspoon confectioners' sugar
3 Granny Smith apples, peeled, cored
    and quartered
10–12 small button mushrooms
1¼ cups dry cider
1¼ cups chicken stock
¾ cup heavy cream
1 teaspoon freshly squeezed lemon juice
1 teaspoon chopped fresh thyme leaves
2 tablespoons chopped fresh parsley
salt and freshly ground black pepper

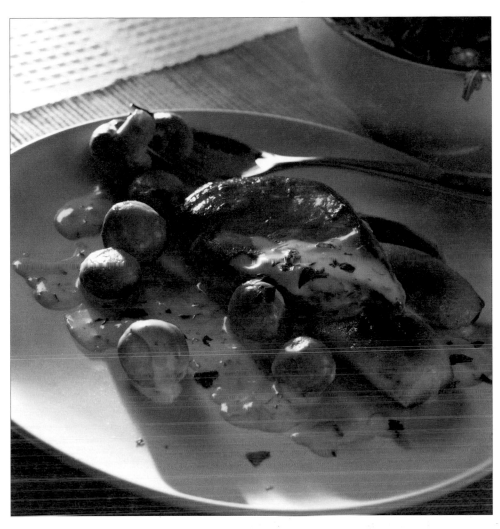

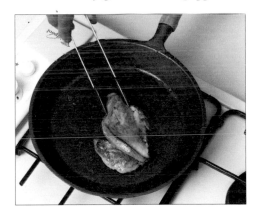

1 Season the pheasant breasts with salt and pepper. Melt 2 tablespoons of the butter in a frying pan and cook the pheasant breasts in batches for about 3 minutes on each side. Transfer to a plate with a slotted spoon.

2 Heat the remaining butter and add the confectioners' sugar and apples. Fry gently for 3 minutes, until the apples are lightly golden. Transfer to the plate with the pheasant breasts.

3 Add the mushrooms to the pan and stir-fry until all the butter has been absorbed.

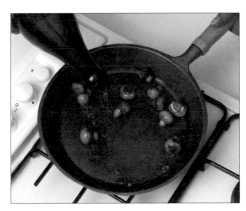

4 Add the cider and boil for 3–5 minutes, until the liquid has almost completely evaporated. Add the chicken stock and simmer until reduced by half. Stir in the cream and heat gently to the boiling point.

5 Return the pheasant breasts and apples to the pan and cook over low heat for 2 minutes. Stir in the lemon juice, thyme and half of the parsley and season with salt and pepper.

6 Arrange the pheasant breasts on four serving plates and pour the sauce over them. Sprinkle with the remaining parsley and serve.

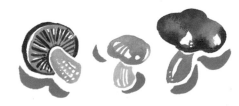

Broiled Spiced Chicken (P)

This dish is delicious served with Fresh Cilantro and Yogurt Dipping Sauce and generous portions of very lightly stir-fried green vegetables, such as snow peas, green beans, broccoli or bok choy.

INGREDIENTS

Serves 4

1 teaspoon coriander seeds
1 teaspoon cumin seeds
2 limes
2 garlic cloves, crushed
¼ cup chopped fresh cilantro
1 small green chili, seeded and
  finely chopped
2 tablespoons light soy sauce
¼ cup sunflower oil
4 boned and skinned chicken breasts,
  about 6 ounces each
green vegetables, to serve

1 Crush the coriander and cumin seeds using a mortar and pestle or coffee grinder.

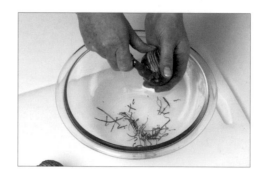

2 Cut the rind from the limes into thin shreds using a zester, avoiding using the pith. Squeeze out the juice from both fruits.

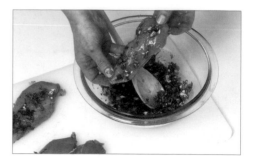

3 Blend the spices, lime rind and juice, garlic, fresh cilantro, chili, soy sauce and oil in a shallow bowl. Add the chicken, turn to coat thoroughly, then cover with plastic wrap and marinate in the refrigerator for 24 hours.

4 Remove the chicken from the marinade. Heat a broiler pan and cook the chicken for 4–6 minutes on each side or until cooked through. Serve with green vegetables.

Moroccan Lamb Kebabs (P)

If you do not have skewers, make small patties instead. The patties can be grilled in exactly the same way as kebabs.

INGREDIENTS

Serves 4

1 pound lean lamb, ground
3 tablespoons grated raw onion
1 tablespoon chopped fresh cilantro
1 tablespoon chopped fresh parsley
1 teaspoon ground cumin
½ teaspoon chili powder
¼ teaspoon ground cinnamon
¼ teaspoon ground ginger
1 tablespoon raisins
1 egg
salt and freshly ground black pepper
grilled lemon halves and sprigs of fresh
  cilantro, to garnish

1 Place the lamb, onion, herbs, spices, raisins, egg and seasoning in a blender or food processor and process for 10–20 seconds or until well blended. Do not overprocess. If you do not have a food processor, lightly beat the egg in a bowl, add the other ingredients and mix thoroughly.

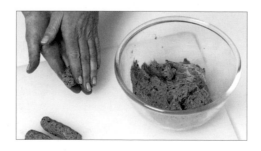

2 Form the mixture into cigar shapes about 4 inches long and place on a plate. Cover with plastic wrap and chill for about 1 hour.

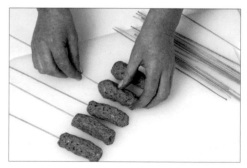

3 Soak 12 wooden skewers in water for 30 minutes. Push a skewer through each of the lamb "cigars," patting the meat around the skewers to retain the shape.

4 Grill or broil for 5–6 minutes, then turn over the kebabs and cook for another 5–6 minutes, until the meat is evenly browned and cooked through. Serve garnished with grilled lemon halves and sprigs of fresh cilantro.

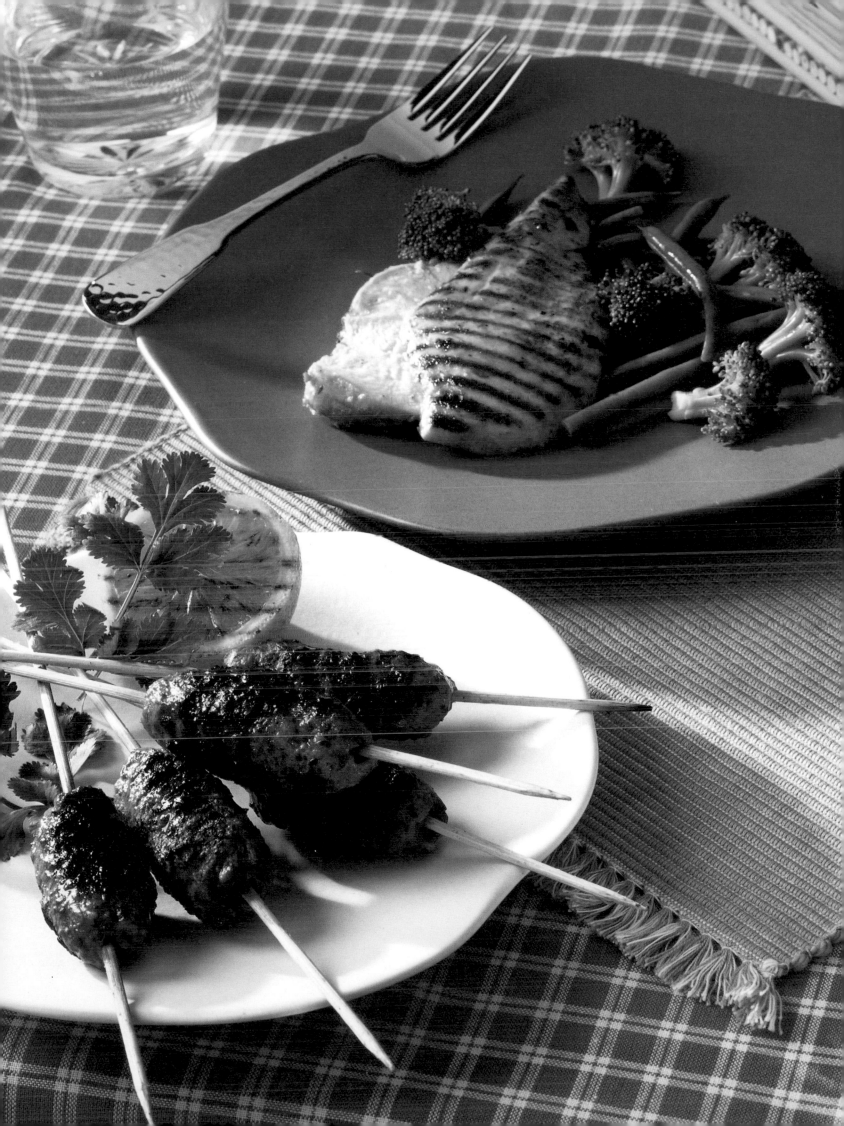

Chicken and Coconut Curry (P)

INGREDIENTS

Serves 4

2 tablespoons peanut oil
1 large onion, finely chopped
2 bay leaves
2 cinnamon sticks
4 cloves
4 cardamom pods, split
1 teaspoon salt
1 teaspoon ground cumin
½ teaspoon ground turmeric
1 teaspoon paprika
1 teaspoon ground coriander
3 garlic cloves, finely chopped
1-inch piece fresh ginger, peeled and
   finely chopped
4 boned and skinned chicken breasts,
   about 8 ounces each, cut into
   ¾-inch pieces
3 tablespoons unsweetened coconut
   cream powder
1¼ cups plain yogurt
½ teaspoon freshly ground black
   pepper
1 cup frozen peas
fresh cilantro leaves, to garnish

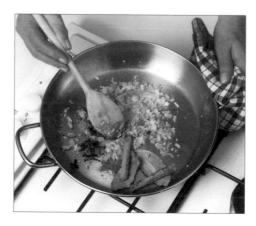

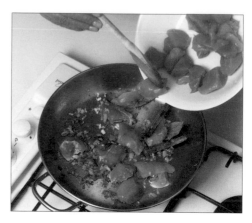

1 Heat the oil in a large heavy saucepan and fry the onion for 5–6 minutes, until transparent, stirring frequently. Add the bay leaves, cinnamon sticks, cloves, cardamom pods, salt, cumin, turmeric, paprika and ground coriander and stir well. Cook over low heat for 2–3 minutes, stirring frequently.

2 Stir in the garlic, ginger and chicken pieces and cook over low heat for 3–4 minutes to brown the chicken.

--- COOK'S TIP ---

Serve with lightly steamed bok choy or snow peas.

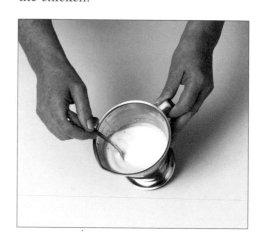

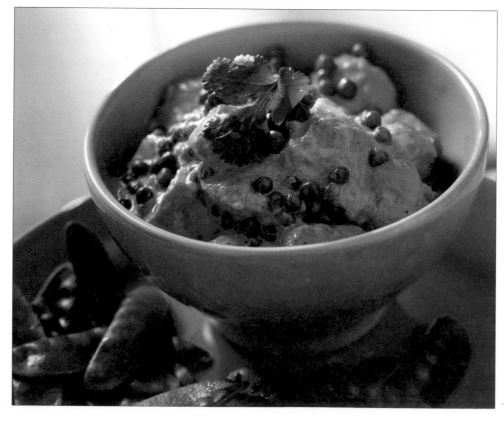

3 Meanwhile, blend the coconut powder with 1¼ cups cold water, stirring thoroughly to remove any lumps. Pour into the pan and cook, uncovered, for about 20 minutes, stirring occasionally until the chicken is cooked and the sauce is thick and well reduced.

4 Stir in the yogurt, black pepper and peas, and simmer for another 10 minutes.

5 Spoon the curry into a warmed serving dish or divide among four serving plates, discarding the bay leaves and cinnamon sticks. Garnish with fresh cilantro and serve.

Poached Chicken with Mustard Mayonnaise (P)

INGREDIENTS

Serves 4

1 leek, trimmed
1 large carrot
1 celery stalk
1 medium onion
1 free-range chicken (3–3½ pounds),
   washed, without giblets
1 tablespoon roughly chopped
   fresh parsley
2 teaspoons roughly chopped
   fresh thyme
6 fresh green peppercorns
mustard mayonnaise, salad greens and
   lightly cooked baby carrots, to serve

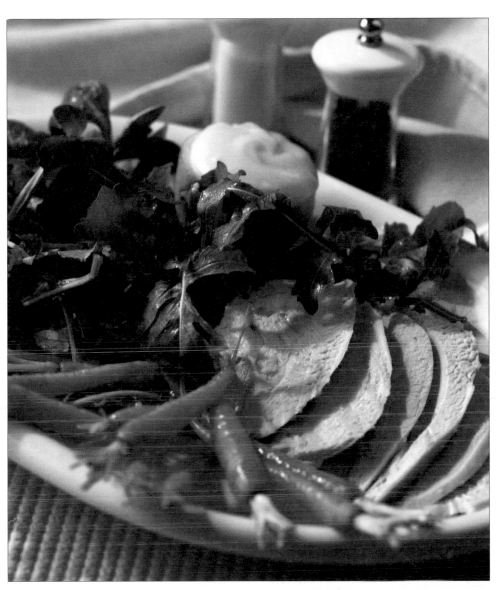

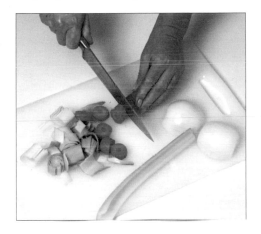

1 Roughly chop the leek, carrot, celery and onion and place in a large saucepan.

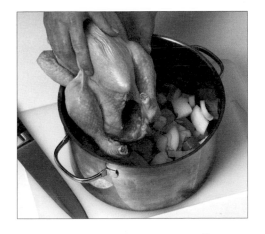

2 Place the chicken on top of the vegetables, cover with water and bring to a boil. Remove any scum that comes to the surface.

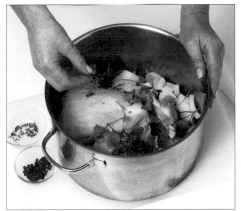

3 Add the herbs and peppercorns. Simmer gently for 1 hour. Remove from the heat and cool in the broth.

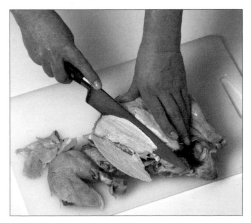

4 Transfer the chicken to a board or plate and carve, removing the skin. Arrange the slices on a serving platter. Serve with mustard mayonnaise, salad greens and lightly cooked baby carrots.

Stir-fried Chicken with Lime and Ginger (P)

Here's a dish that can be prepared in advance and then cooked in minutes. Hoisin sauce is a thick, sweet soy bean sauce available at most supermarkets.

INGREDIENTS

Serves 4

2 tablespoons hoisin sauce
2 tablespoons honey
juice of 1 lime
1½ pounds boned and skinned
   chicken fillet, cut into thin strips
6 tablespoons peanut oil
1 carrot, cut into thin strips
2-inch piece fresh ginger, peeled and
   cut into thin strips
2 tablespoons light soy sauce
1 lime, thinly sliced

1 Blend the hoisin sauce, honey and lime juice in a large bowl and add the chicken strips, stirring well. Cover and place in the refrigerator for 1–2 hours to marinate.

2 Heat the oil in a wok or large frying pan until very hot and almost smoking, and then stir-fry the carrot and ginger until crisp and golden. Transfer with a slotted spoon to a plate lined with paper towels.

--- VARIATION ---

This is also delicious with stir-fried broccoli, bok choy and toasted almonds.

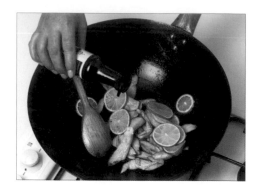

3 Pour half the oil out of the pan, then add the chicken and stir-fry for 3–5 minutes, until the chicken is cooked through and brown. Add the soy sauce and lime slices, stirring constantly. Serve with the shreds of fried ginger and carrot scattered on top of the chicken.

Crispy Duck Breasts with Bok Choy (P)

If possible, use wild duck for this recipe. It is in season from the beginning of September to the end of January and is much leaner and tastier than the more fatty farmyard ducks. Bok choy, also known as mustard greens, is a type of Chinese cabbage.

INGREDIENTS

Serves 4

4 duck breasts, about 6 ounces each
1 pound bok choy
4 scallions, trimmed
3 tablespoons light soy sauce
2 tablespoons lemon juice
2 teaspoons English mustard powder,
   blended with 2 teaspoons cold water
½-inch piece fresh ginger, peeled and
   finely shredded
salt and freshly ground black pepper

1 Prick the skin of the duck breasts all over with a fork and rub well with salt and pepper. Heat a heavy frying pan, place the breasts in it skin side down and fry undisturbed for 12–14 minutes over very low heat.

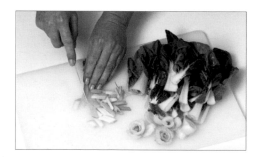

2 Meanwhile, remove any tough bok choy stalks and cut the scallions into diagonal 1-inch lengths. Blanch the bok choy and scallions in lightly salted water for about 1 minute or until the bok choy wilts. Then immerse in very cold water for 30 seconds and drain well. Squeeze out excess water and fluff out the leaves.

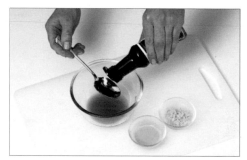

3 Combine the soy sauce, lemon juice, mustard and ginger in a large bowl, add the bok choy and toss to mix. Place the leaves in four bowls.

4 Turn over the duck breasts and fry on the other side for 3 minutes. Preheat the broiler and broil the duck, skin side up, for 2–3 minutes, until the skin is brown and crisp.

5 Let the meat stand for about 5 minutes before carving, then slice each breast in half horizontally or into 4–6 pieces. Serve with the bok choy.

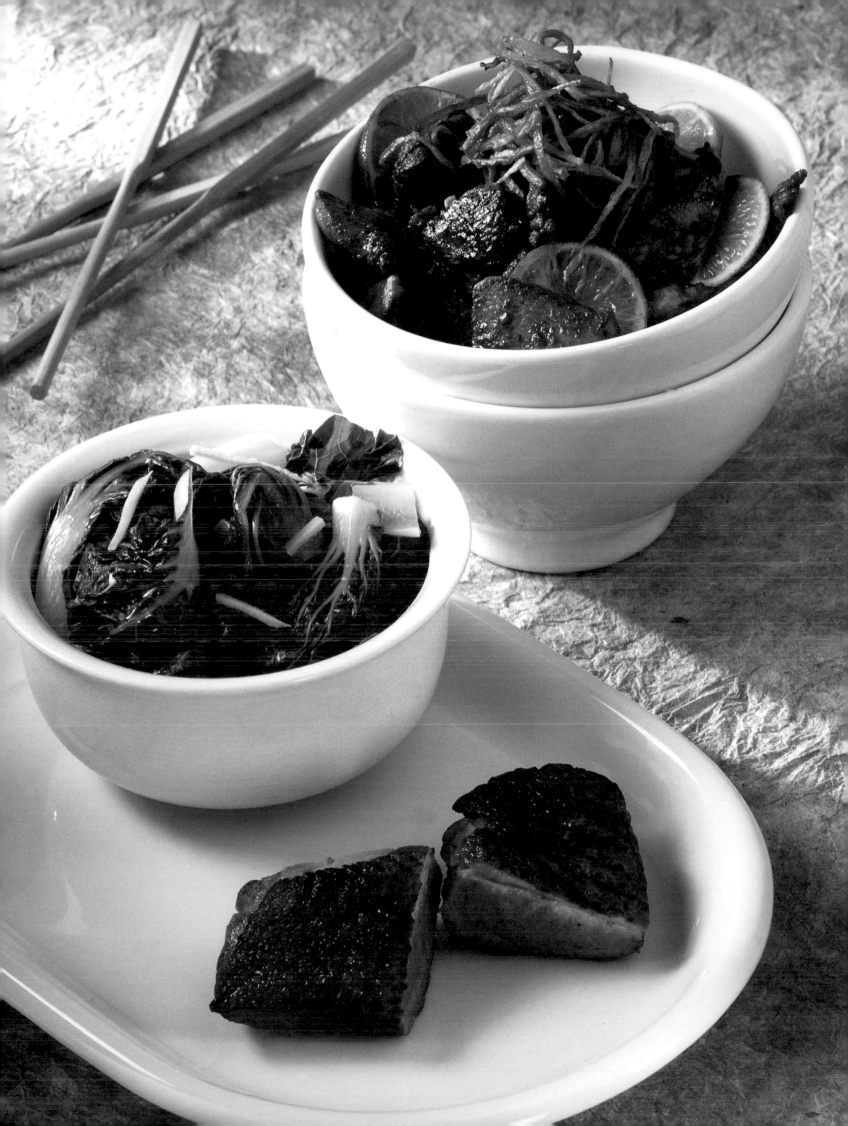

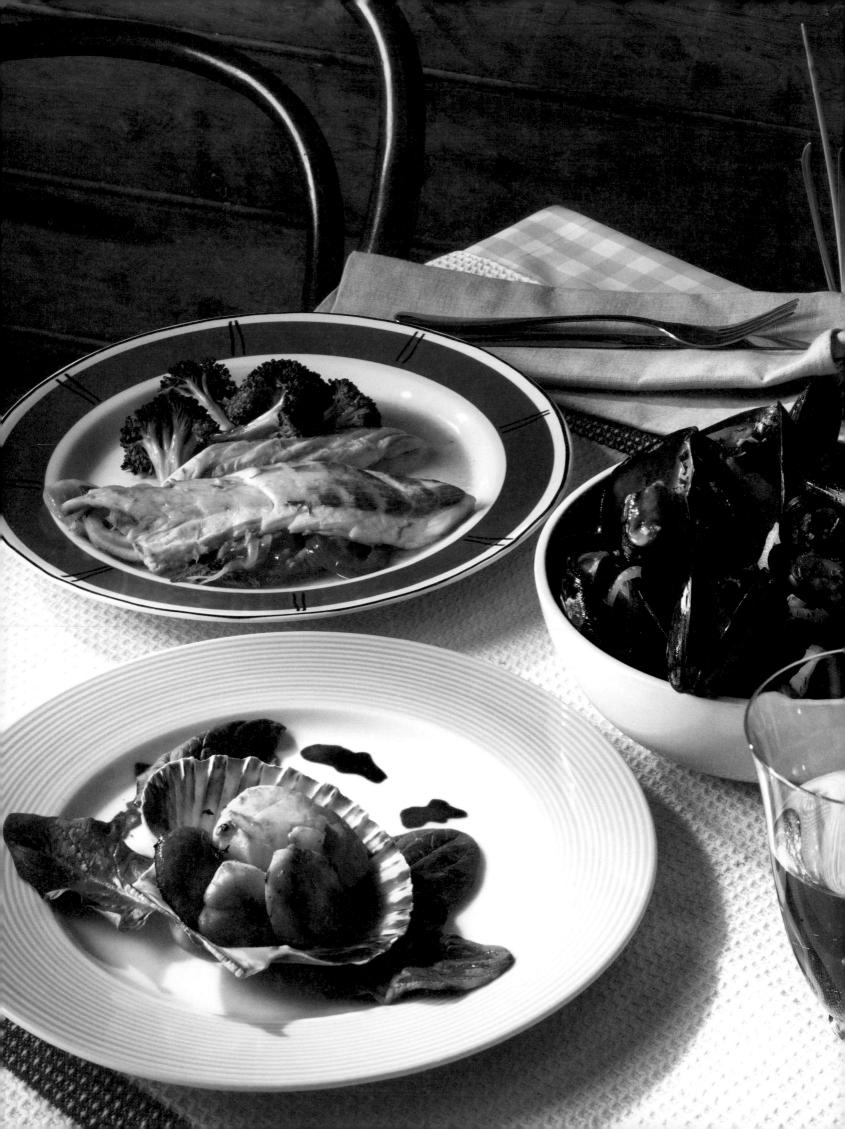

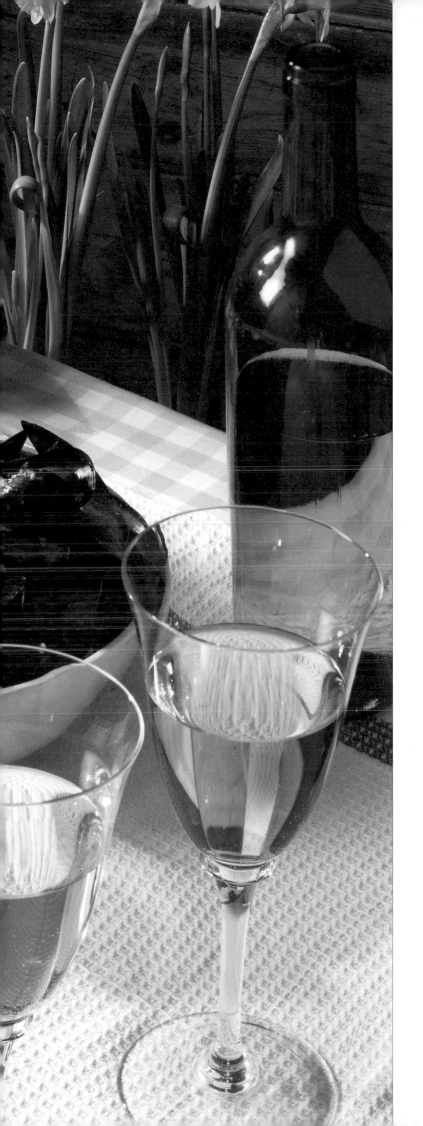

FISH AND SEAFOOD

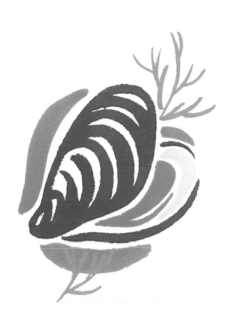

Although most fish and seafood are available all year round, many varieties have a natural season when they are plentiful and have the best flavor. You don't need masses of other ingredients to make fish dishes as delicious as roasted cod with a smooth, fresh tomato sauce or broiled salmon served with a super-easy yogurt sauce subtly flavored with fresh mint and cucumber. Whole sea bass baked "en papillote" is simplicity itself—the paper parcel conserves all the aromatic juices of the fish, which are released only as you serve the fish.

Roasted Cod with Fresh Tomato Sauce (P)

Really fresh cod has a sweet, delicate flavor and a pure white flaky flesh. Served with an aromatic tomato sauce, it provides a nutritious meal.

INGREDIENTS

Serves 4

12 ounces fresh ripe plum tomatoes
5 tablespoons olive oil
½ teaspoon superfine sugar
2 strips of orange rind
1 fresh thyme sprig
6 fresh basil leaves
2 pounds fresh cod fillet with skin
salt and freshly ground black pepper
steamed green beans, to serve

1 Preheat the oven to 450°F. Roughly chop the tomatoes.

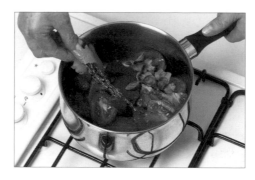

2 Heat 1 tablespoon of the olive oil in a heavy saucepan, add the tomatoes, sugar, orange rind, thyme and basil and simmer for 5 minutes, until the tomatoes are soft.

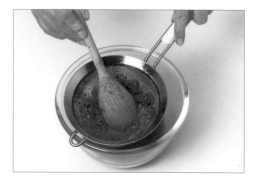

3 Press the tomato mixture through a fine sieve, discarding the tomato skins and seeds, orange rind and hard pieces of thyme. Pour into a small saucepan and heat gently.

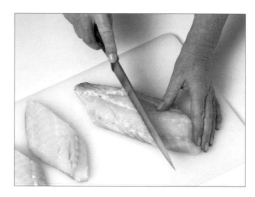

4 Scale the cod fillet and cut on the diagonal into four equal pieces. Season well with salt and pepper.

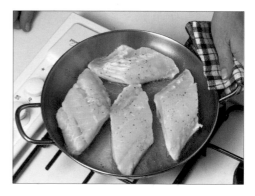

5 Heat the remaining oil in a clean heavy frying pan and fry the cod, skin side down, until the skin is crisp. Place the fish on a greased baking sheet, skin side up, and roast for 8–10 minutes, until the fish is cooked through. Serve the fish on the steamed green beans with the tomato sauce drizzled over it.

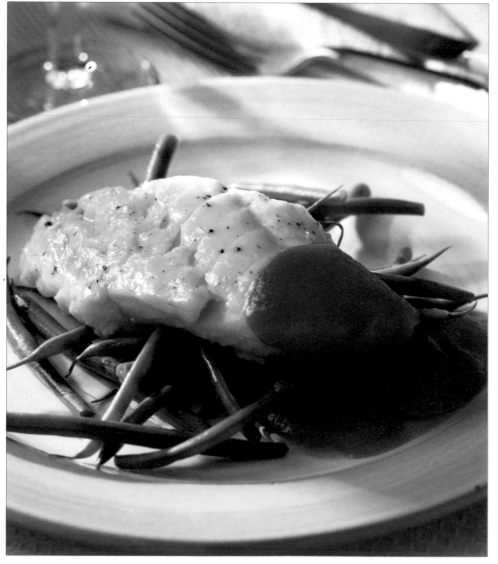

Haddock in Spinach Parcels with Pepper Purée (P)

This recipe really deserves a freshly made fish stock, but stock made from vegetable bouillon powder is preferable to most stock cubes. It is delicious served with a bell pepper purée.

INGREDIENTS

Serves 4

1 tablespoon olive oil
1 small shallot, sliced
2 garlic cloves, sliced
2 yellow bell peppers, chopped
1 fresh thyme sprig
2½ cups fish stock
¼ cup heavy cream
4 fresh haddock fillets, about 6 ounces
    each, skinned
8 large spinach leaves, blanched
salt and freshly ground black pepper

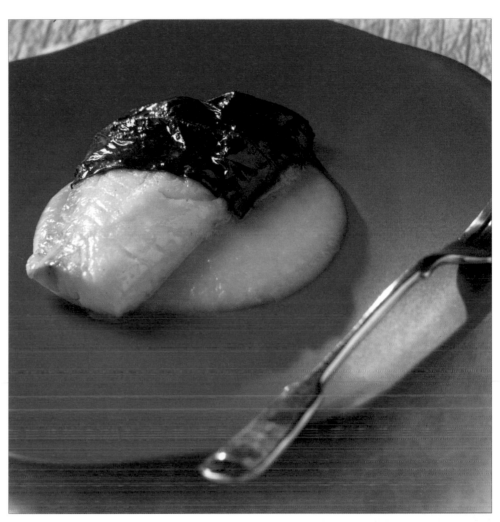

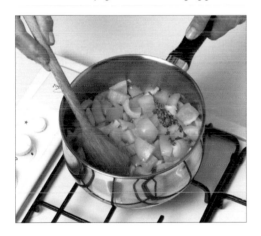

1 Heat the oil in a heavy pan and fry the shallot and garlic for 3 minutes, stirring frequently. Add the peppers, thyme and 2 cups of the fish stock. Season with salt and pepper, then simmer for 15 minutes, until the peppers are tender.

COOK'S TIP

To blanch spinach leaves, place them in a colander and pour boiling water over them. Plunge them immediately into ice-cold water to set the color.

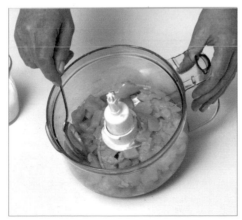

2 Place the pepper mixture in a blender or food processor, then process until smooth. Stir in the cream, then pour into a clean saucepan and heat gently to warm through.

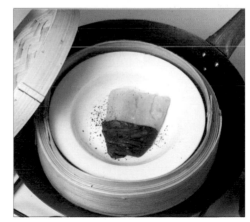

3 Meanwhile, half-wrap each fish fillet in two of the blanched spinach leaves. Place the remaining stock in a pan and bring to a boil. Place the fish parcels in a steamer, season, then set them over the stock and steam for 4 minutes. Arrange the fish parcels on four warmed serving plates and serve with the warm sauce.

Stuffed Sardines with Fresh Rosemary (P)

If fresh sardines are not available, choose four small herrings or two mackerel—they are also delicious cooked this way.

INGREDIENTS

Serves 4
1 tablespoon olive oil
3 pounds fresh sardines
1 large sprig fresh rosemary
3 tablespoons chopped fresh parsley
1 shallot, finely chopped
1 cup pine nuts
2 garlic cloves, finely chopped
juice and finely grated rind of
    1 large lemon
salt and freshly ground black pepper
lemon wedges and sprigs of fresh
    rosemary, to garnish

1 Preheat the oven to 375°F and brush an ovenproof dish with a little of the olive oil. Remove the heads of the sardines and split each one down the belly.

2 Place the fish on a cutting board, cut side down, and gently but firmly press down on the backbone. Turn them over and ease out the backbone. Wash the fish well in salted water and pat dry.

3 Pull the rosemary leaves off of the stem and chop finely. Place in a bowl and mix with the parsley, shallot, pine nuts and garlic.

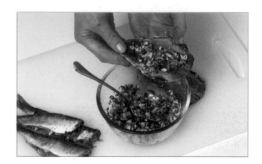

4 Season the fish inside and out with salt and pepper and place a spoonful or two of stuffing inside each one. Press the sides around the stuffing and place each fish in the baking dish.

5 Sprinkle on the remaining olive oil and bake for 30 minutes. Just before serving, squeeze on the lemon juice and sprinkle with the lemon rind. Garnish with lemon wedges and sprigs of rosemary.

Fried Monkfish with Homemade Tapenade (P)

INGREDIENTS

Serves 3–4
1 pound fresh monkfish fillet
2 tablespoons olive oil
salt and freshly ground black pepper
chopped fresh parsley and diced red
    bell pepper, to garnish

For the tapenade
1 pound black olives, pitted
1 tablespoon capers, drained and rinsed
1 can (2 ounces) anchovy fillets,
    drained and diced
1 tablespoon Dijon mustard
10 fresh basil leaves, roughly torn
4 garlic cloves, crushed
about ½ cup extra virgin olive oil
1 tablespoon brandy
½ teaspoon freshly ground
    black pepper

1 To make the tapenade, place all the ingredients in a blender or food processor and process until the mixture is well blended but still has a little texture, adding a little extra olive oil if necessary. You will need about half of the mixture for this recipe—store the remainder in the refrigerator in an airtight jar.

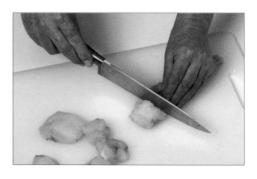

2 Cut the fish into rounds about 1 inch thick. Season with salt and pepper.

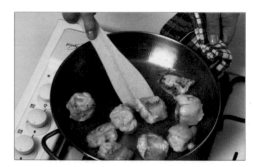

3 Heat the olive oil in a heavy frying pan and fry the fish on one side for 2 minutes. Turn the fish over and cook for another 1 minute.

4 Place a generous spoonful of tapenade in the center of four serving plates and arrange the fish around each mound. Sprinkle with parsley and diced red pepper and serve.

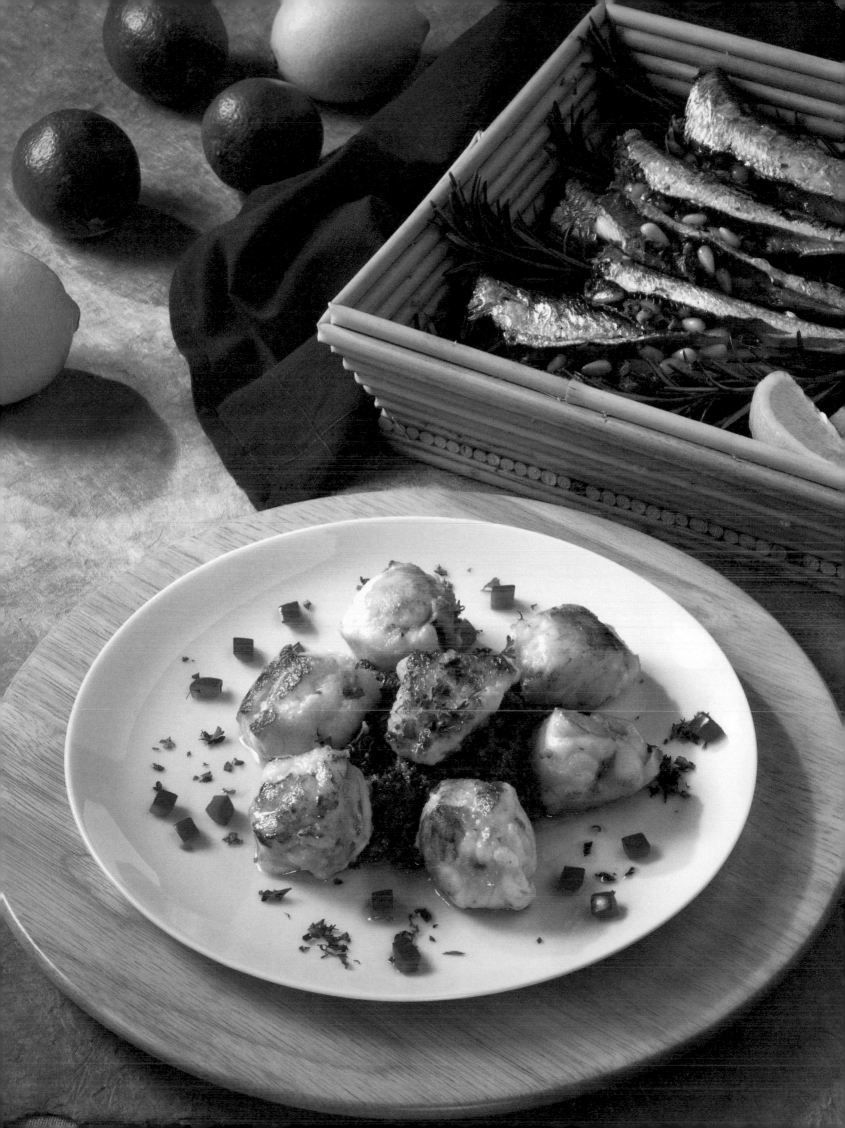

Whole Sea Bass en Papillote (P)

Sea bass is also known as sea wolf, sea dace or sea perch and has delicate pink flesh and a light sweet smell. Cooking in parchment paper means the fish retains its flavor. Mullet and bream can be cooked in the same way.

Ingredients

Serves 4

fresh whole sea bass (3–3½ pounds),
   cleaned, scaled and head removed
5 fresh mint sprigs
½ lemon, sliced
2 shallots, finely sliced
2 fresh plum tomatoes, sliced
3 tablespoons olive oil
salt and freshly ground black pepper
steamed broccoli, to serve

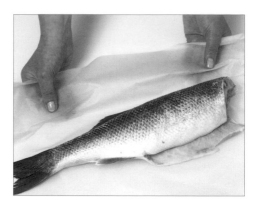

1 Preheat the oven to 350°F. Wash and dry the fish and place on a double piece of parchment paper, large enough to wrap the fish completely.

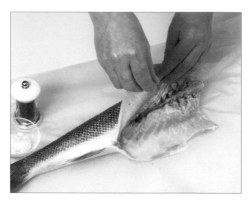

2 Season the fish inside and out with salt and pepper.

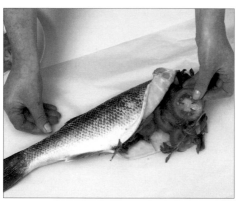

3 Tuck the fresh mint sprigs, lemon slices, shallots and tomato slices inside the fish and drizzle the olive oil over its back.

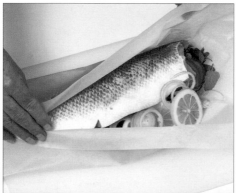

4 Fold the paper over the fish and double-fold the three open edges.

5 Place the fish on a baking sheet and bake for 40–50 minutes, until cooked through. Cut the package open with scissors and serve the fish with steamed broccoli.

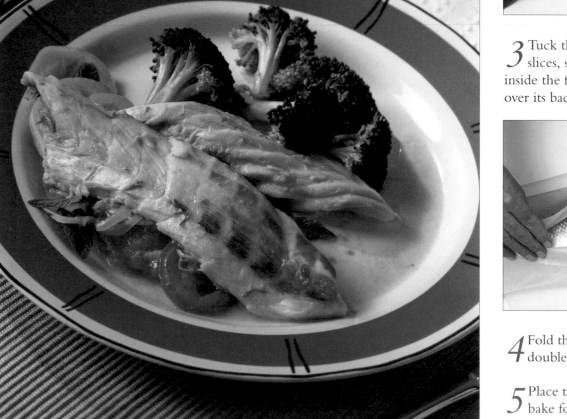

Salmon with Yogurt and Mint Dressing (P)

Salmon is a very rich fish and is delicious, broiled and served with this light and delicate sauce. A mixed green leaf and herb salad makes a perfect accompaniment.

INGREDIENTS

Serves 4
½ large cucumber
6 fresh mint leaves
⅔ cup plain yogurt
fresh salmon fillet (1½ pounds), middle cut with skin
1 teaspoon olive oil
salt and freshly ground black pepper
mint sprigs, to garnish
fresh spinach leaves, to serve

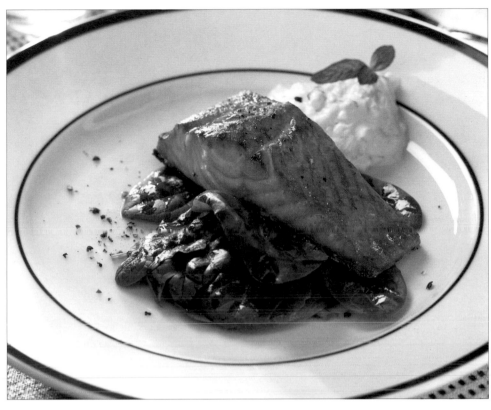

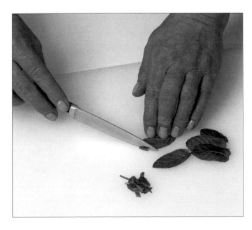

1 Peel the cucumber, slice in half lengthwise and remove the seeds.

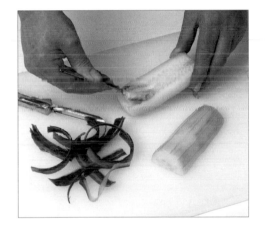

2 Grate the cucumber into a sieve, salt lightly and drain for about 30 minutes. Chop the mint leaves.

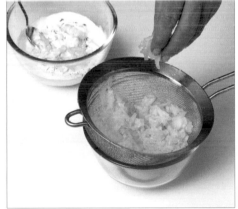

3 Place the chopped mint leaves in a bowl with the yogurt. Squeeze out any excess juice from the cucumber and stir into the bowl with the yogurt and mint. Season with black pepper.

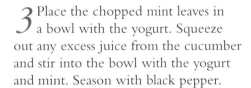

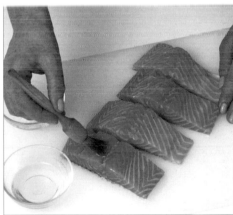

4 Preheat the broiler until medium hot. Scale the salmon if the fishmonger has not already done this, and check for any bones. Cut the salmon into four pieces, brush with the olive oil and season with a little salt.

5 Broil the fish for 3 minutes, skin side up, then carefully turn over the fish and broil for about 2 minutes on the other side. The skin should be brown and crisp. Serve on a bed of spinach with the yogurt and cucumber dressing. Garnish with sprigs of mint and grind on some black pepper.

Butterflied Mediterranean Shrimp (P)

Skewered shrimp, marinated in a fiery herb dressing, then grilled until pink and tender, make a delicious light lunch or summer supper dish.

INGREDIENTS

Serves 4
32 jumbo shrimp, peeled
2 garlic cloves, finely chopped
6 tablespoons finely chopped
  fresh parsley
chopped leaves of 1 fresh
  rosemary sprig
pinch of dried chili flakes
juice of 2 fresh limes
2 tablespoons olive oil
salt and freshly ground black pepper
green salad, to serve

1 Wash the shrimp in salted water, remove their heads and shells, then remove the black thread that runs along the back of the shrimp. To butterfly the shrimp, cut along the back, without completely cutting through, then carefully fan out.

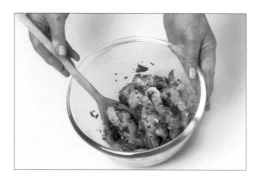

2 Blend the garlic, parsley, rosemary, chili flakes, lime juice, olive oil, and seasoning in a bowl. Add the shrimp, stir well and let marinate for 1 hour.

3 Meanwhile, soak 32 wooden skewers in warm water for at least 30 minutes.

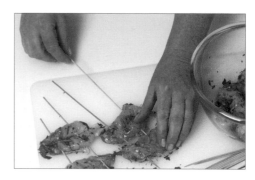

4 Preheat the broiler until very hot. Thread 2 shrimp onto each pair of skewers and broil for 2–3 minutes, until each side has turned bright pink. Remove the shrimp from the skewers and serve with green salad.

Seared Scallops with Lemon and Thyme (P)

Scallop shells make attractive little dishes and most good fishmongers will sell you the scallops and shells together. Make sure the shells are well scrubbed and clean before using.

INGREDIENTS

Serves 4
¼ cup olive oil
2 garlic cloves, finely chopped
4 fresh thyme sprigs
1 bay leaf
1 tablespoon chopped fresh parsley
16 fresh scallops, rinsed
1 shallot, finely chopped
1 tablespoon balsamic vinegar
2 tablespoons lemon juice
⅔ cup chicken or vegetable stock
salt and freshly ground black pepper
24 baby spinach leaves, to garnish

1 Blend the olive oil, garlic, thyme, bay leaf and parsley in a shallow bowl. Add the scallops and let marinate in a cool place for 1 hour.

2 Heat a heavy frying pan until smoking. Remove the scallops from the marinade and sear for about 30 seconds on each side to seal in their juices. Transfer the scallops to a plate and keep warm.

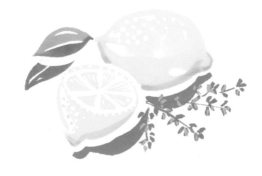

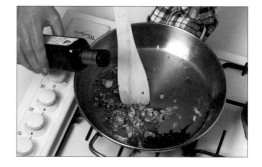

3 Add the marinade to the pan, then add the shallot and balsamic vinegar, lemon juice and stock. Cook over high heat for 5 minutes, until the stock is well reduced. Discard the bay leaf and season with salt and pepper.

4 Arrange 6 spinach leaves around each scallop shell in the center of four serving plates, place 4 scallops in each shell and pour on the juices.

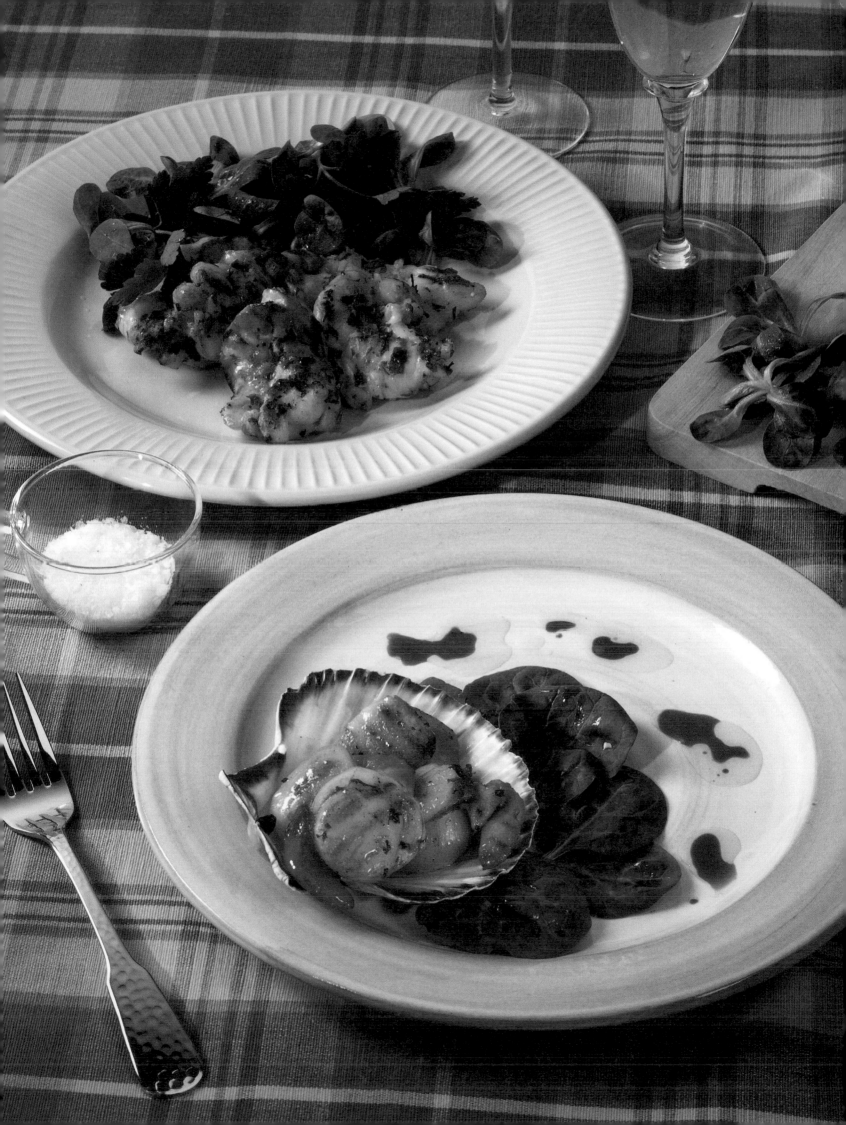

Mussels in Fennel and White Wine (P)

INGREDIENTS

Serves 4

3–3½ pounds fresh mussels
3 shallots
3 garlic cloves
1 small fennel bulb
1 tablespoon olive oil
1¼ cups dry white wine
1 tablespoon chopped fresh parsley
juice of ½ lemon
salt and freshly ground black pepper
chopped fresh parsley, to garnish

— COOK'S TIP —

After you have washed the mussels, give any that are open a sharp tap, and if they refuse to close, discard them. Conversely, any mussels that remain closed after cooking should also be thrown away.

1 Scrub the mussels thoroughly in several changes of water (see Cook's Tip) and pull off the beards. Set the mussels aside.

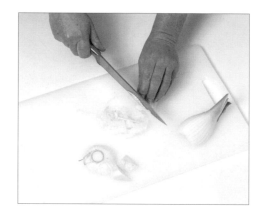

2 Finely chop the shallots and garlic. Remove the root from the fennel and slice finely.

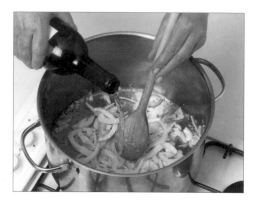

3 Heat the oil in a heavy pan and fry the shallots, fennel and garlic for 1 minute, stirring constantly. Add the wine and simmer for 5 minutes.

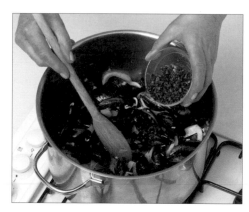

4 Add the mussels and parsley, cover with a tight-fitting lid and cook for 4 minutes, shaking the pan occasionally. Remove the lid and check that all the mussels are open.

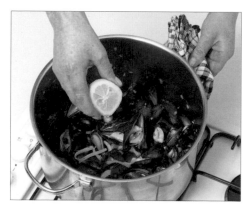

5 Squeeze in the lemon juice, then season to taste. Divide the mussels among four large bowls. Pour the liquid over the mussels and sprinkle with chopped parsley.

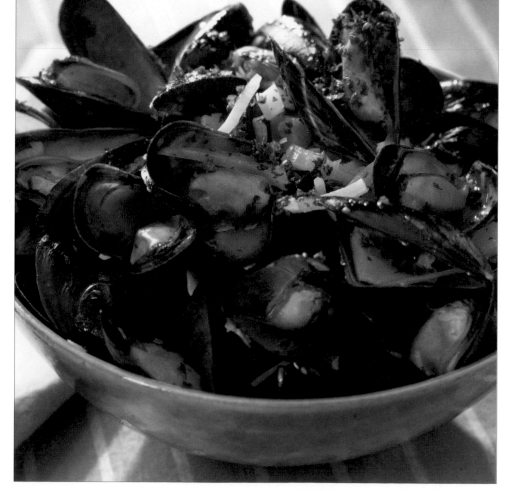

Seafarer's Stew (P)

Any variety of firm fish may be used in this recipe, but be sure to use smoked haddock as well; it is essential for its distinctive flavor.

INGREDIENTS

Serves 4

naturally smoked haddock fillet
   (8 ounces), uncolored
fresh monkfish fillet (8 ounces)
20 fresh mussels, scrubbed
2 strips bacon (optional)
1 tablespoon olive oil
1 shallot, finely chopped
4 carrots, coarsely grated
²/₃ cup light or heavy cream or
   half-and-half
12 cooked peeled jumbo shrimp
salt and freshly ground black pepper
2 tablespoons chopped fresh parsley,
   to garnish

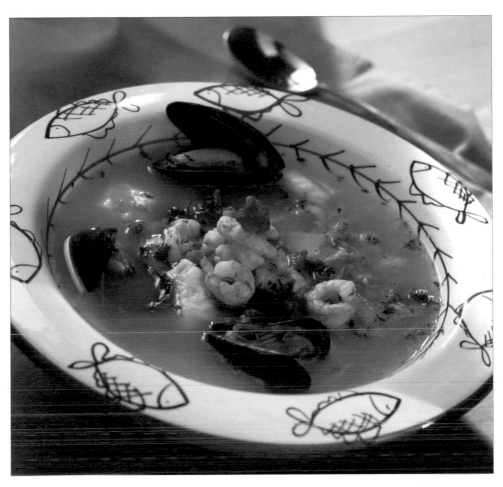

1 In a large heavy pan, simmer the haddock and monkfish in 5 cups water for 5 minutes, then add the mussels and cover the pan with a lid.

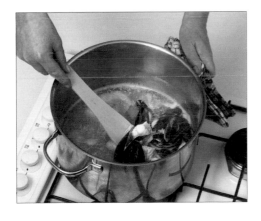

2 Cook for another 5 minutes or until all the mussels have opened. Discard any that have not. Drain, reserving the liquid. Return the liquid to the rinsed pan and set aside.

3 Flake the haddock coarsely, removing any skin and bones, then cut the monkfish into large chunks. Cut the bacon, if using, into strips.

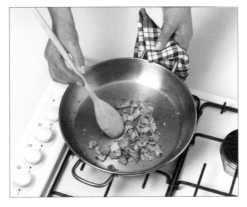

4 Heat the oil in a heavy frying pan and fry the shallot and bacon for 3–4 minutes or until the shallot is soft and the bacon lightly brown. Add to the strained fish broth, bring to a boil, then add the grated carrots and cook for 10 minutes.

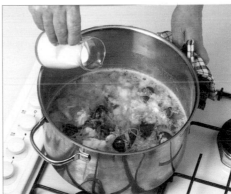

5 Stir in the cream with the haddock, monkfish, mussels and shrimp and heat gently, without boiling. Season and serve in large bowls, garnished with parsley.

COOK'S TIP

The advantage of using heavy cream is that the liquid will not curdle if you do accidentally let it boil.

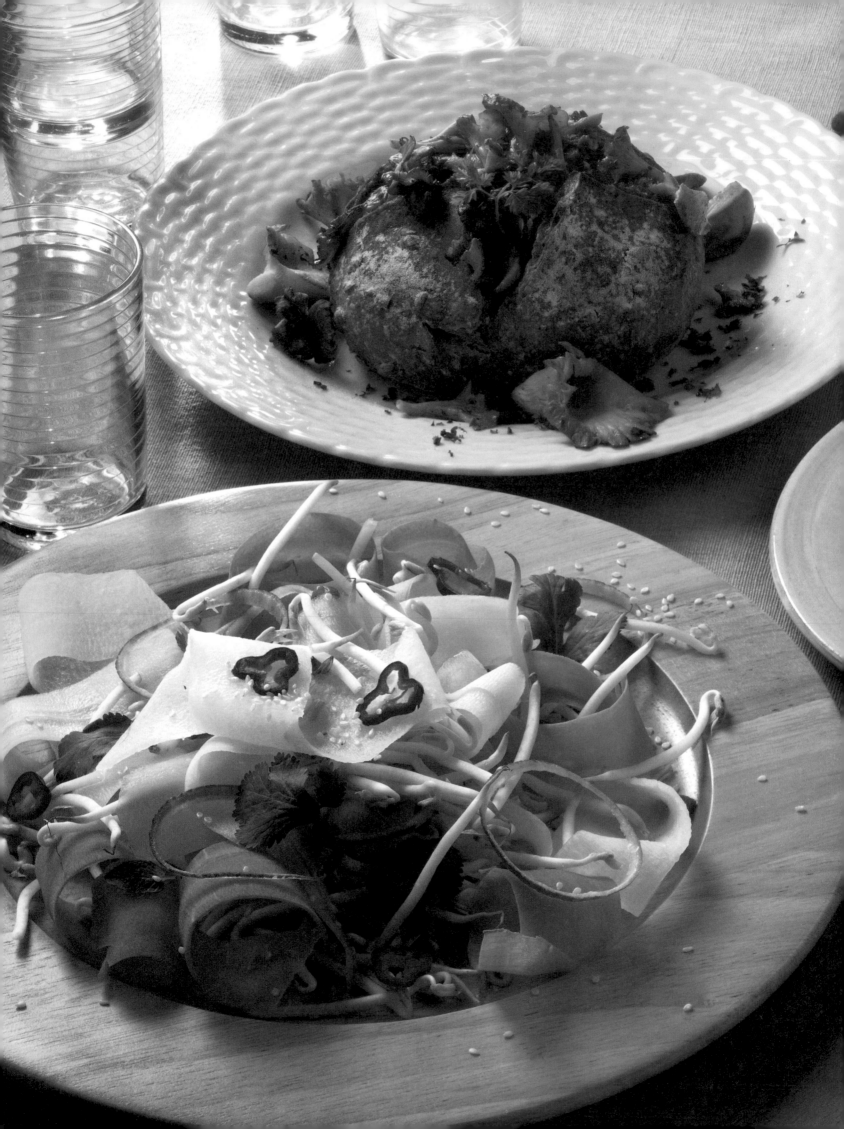

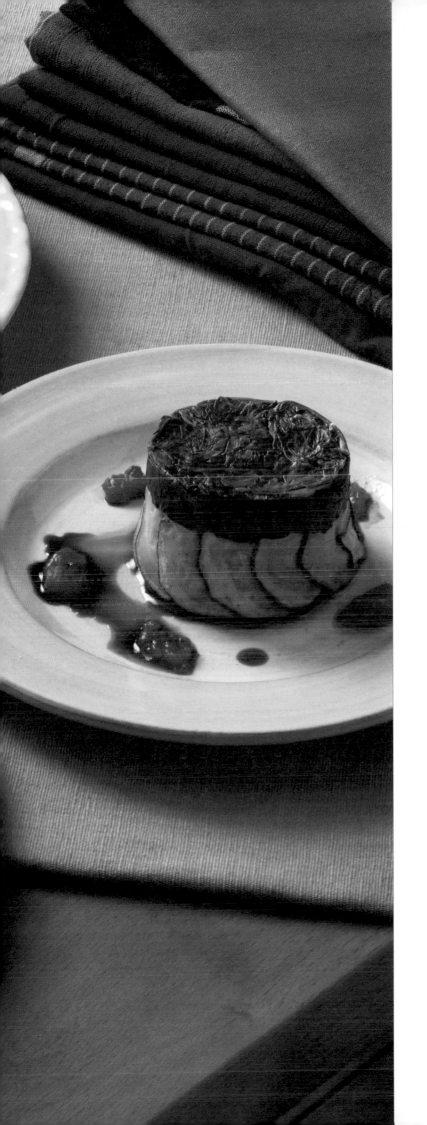

VEGETABLES AND SALADS

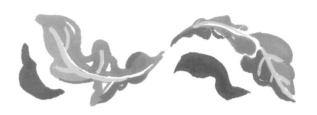

Vegetables and salads are vital to healthy eating and should be considered an important part of each meal and not just an occasional accompaniment. For the finest flavor, choose organic and seasonal varieties whenever possible. A Mixed Mushroom Sandwich is a meal in itself served in a hollowed-out whole-wheat roll and accompanied by lots of fresh salad. Celeriac, Turnip and Carrot Purée is delicious to mop up the juices of fish or game, and makes a nutritious meal on its own served with nutty brown rice generously scattered with toasted hazelnuts.

Winter Vegetable Ragout (S)

INGREDIENTS

Serves 4

2 tablespoons extra virgin olive oil
1 onion, finely chopped
1 ounce dried porcini mushrooms,
  rinsed well, then soaked in 1¼ cups
  hot water for 10 minutes
2 garlic cloves, finely chopped
1 fresh thyme sprig
2 bay leaves
4 carrots, cut into 2-inch sticks
1 celery stalk, sliced
1 small cauliflower, broken
  into florets
2 parsnips, cut into 2-inch sticks
2 large potatoes, cubed
1 cup button mushrooms
1 cup baby Brussels sprouts
salt and freshly ground black pepper
2 tablespoons each chopped fresh
  parsley and tarragon, to garnish

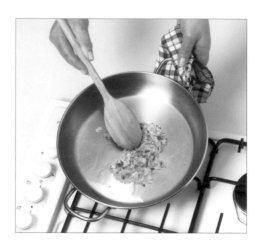

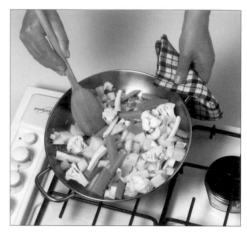

1 Heat the olive oil in a large heavy frying pan and fry the onion for 4–5 minutes until golden brown. Drain the mushrooms, reserving the soaking liquid.

2 Add the garlic, thyme, bay leaves, carrots, celery, cauliflower, parsnips and potatoes. Stir well and cook for 2 minutes.

3 Strain the mushroom liquid and add to the pan with the porcini mushrooms. Cover and cook gently for 10 minutes.

4 Add the button mushrooms and Brussels sprouts and cook for another 5 minutes until all of the vegetables are tender. Taste and adjust the seasoning, then serve, with the chopped parsley and tarragon sprinkled over the top.

--- COOK'S TIP ---

Turn the ragout into a pie by covering it with a thick layer of mashed potatoes. Bake at 350°F for another 30 minutes, until the potatoes are golden brown.

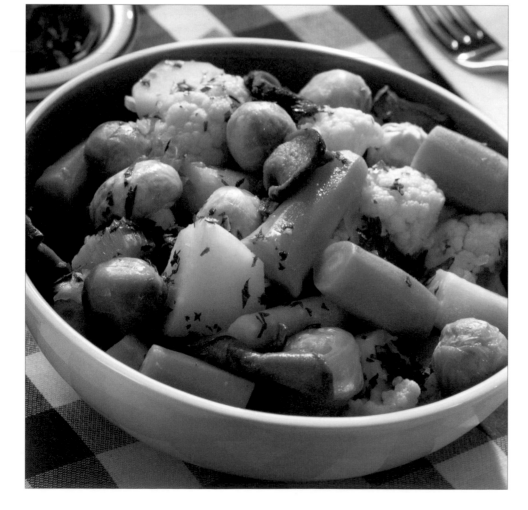

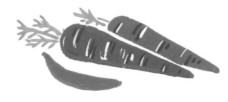

Almost-dry Roasted Vegetables (N)

This is a delicious if rather slow method of cooking vegetables, but they retain all their juicy flavor. Serve them with pasta, hot toast or Grilled Polenta as a starch main course.

INGREDIENTS

Serves 4
1 eggplant
2 zucchini
1 yellow bell pepper
1 red bell pepper
4 garlic cloves
1 sweet red onion
1 small fennel bulb
20 small asparagus spears
10 fresh basil leaves, roughly torn
3 tablespoons extra virgin olive oil
1 tablespoon balsamic vinegar
salt and freshly ground black pepper
sprigs of basil, to garnish

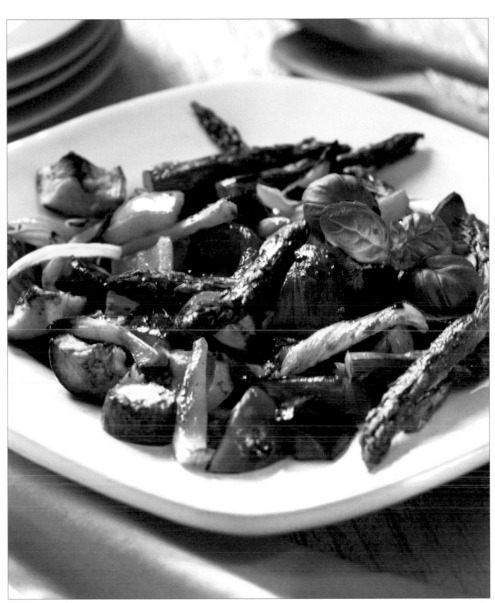

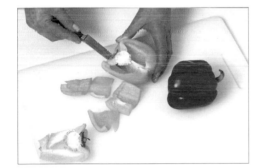

1 Preheat the oven to 475°F. Cut the eggplant and zucchini into ¼-inch slices. Halve the peppers, discard the seeds and core, then cut them into chunks.

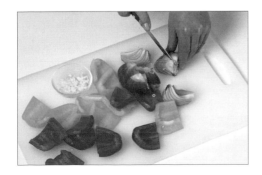

2 Finely chop the garlic and cut the onion into eight wedges.

3 Remove the root from the fennel and slice into 1-inch strips.

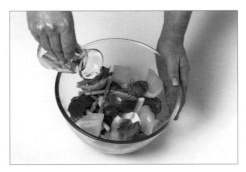

4 Place all the vegetables in a bowl, add the basil, then stir in the olive oil. Season with salt and pepper and combine well.

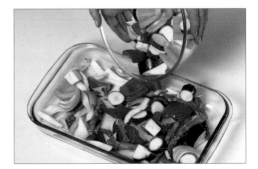

5 Transfer the vegetables to a shallow roasting pan and roast for 30–40 minutes, until the vegetables are brown on the edges. Let cool, then sprinkle with the balsamic vinegar and serve garnished with sprigs of basil.

Celeriac, Turnip and Carrot Purée (N)

This sophisticated, subtly colored combination of root vegetables is delicious with both meat and fish. Parsnips and rutabaga have stronger flavors and are excellent with pheasant and pork.

INGREDIENTS

Serves 4
1 celeriac
4 turnips
4 carrots
1 small shallot
2 tablespoons butter
1 tablespoon light cream or half-and-half
1/4 teaspoon freshly grated nutmeg
salt and freshly ground black pepper
fresh chives, to garnish

1 Peel the celeriac and peel or scrape the turnips if necessary.

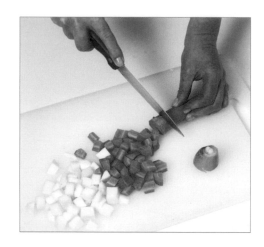

2 Cut the celeriac, turnips and carrots into bite-size pieces and finely chop the shallot. Place in a pan of very lightly salted boiling water. Cook for 8 minutes, until tender but still firm.

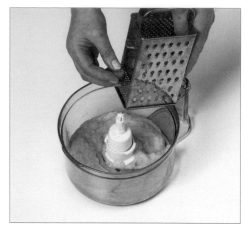

3 Drain in a colander and place in a blender or food processor with the butter and cream. Process to a fine purée, then season with salt, pepper and nutmeg. Spoon directly into four serving bowls. Garnish with fresh chives and serve immediately.

Stir-fried Green Beans with Ginger (N)

Green beans keep their crunchy texture even after cooking and may be served cold as an alternative salad or as a tasty light appetizer.

INGREDIENTS

Serves 4
1/2-inch piece fresh ginger
1 pound fresh green beans
2 tablespoons olive oil
1/2 teaspoon black mustard seeds
1/4 cup water
1/2 teaspoon ground cumin
1/4 teaspoon ground turmeric
2 tablespoons chopped fresh cilantro
1 teaspoon salt
1 teaspoon lemon juice
freshly ground black pepper
shreds of fried ginger, to garnish

1 Peel the ginger and cut into very fine strips. Trim the beans and cut in half.

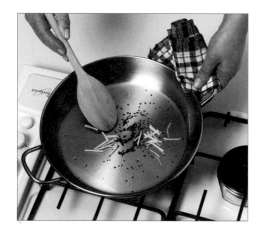

2 Heat the olive oil in a large frying pan, wok or flameproof casserole and sauté the mustard seeds and ginger until the seeds crackle.

3 Add the beans and stir-fry over medium heat for 5 minutes.

4 Add the water, cover the pan and simmer for 3 minutes. Remove the lid and simmer until almost all the water has evaporated, then add the cumin, turmeric, cilantro and salt.

5 Continue cooking until the beans are tender but crisp, and the water has completely evaporated. Add the lemon juice, season with black pepper and garnish with shreds of ginger. Serve immediately.

COOK'S TIP

Be careful not to let the beans overcook or they will lose their delicious crunchy texture.

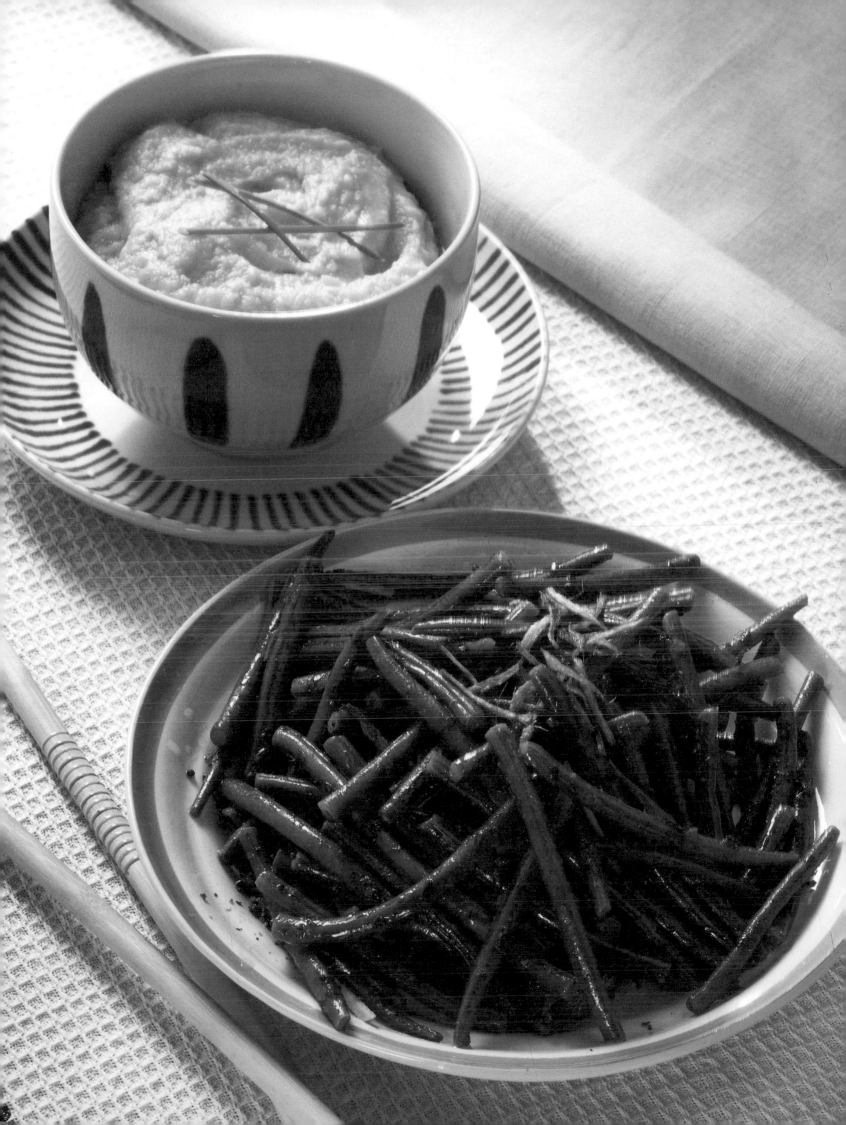

Mixed Mushroom Sandwiches (S)

Nothing can match the flavor of freshly picked wild mushrooms; the next best thing is to combine several different cultivated types. If possible, choose organically grown mushrooms, which have a richer flavor.

INGREDIENTS

Serves 4

2 garlic cloves
1 shallot
1 pound mixed mushrooms, such as oyster, button and cepes
5 tablespoons olive oil
2 tablespoons chopped fresh chervil
2 tablespoons chopped fresh parsley
chopped leaves of 1 fresh rosemary sprig
salt and freshly ground black pepper
sprigs of fresh chervil, to garnish
4 rolls, to serve

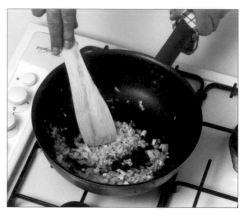

1 Finely chop the garlic and shallot. Wipe the mushrooms, carefully removing any dirt and discarding any very tough stems. Slice the larger mushrooms and halve the smaller ones.

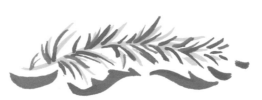

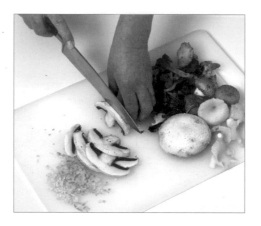

2 Heat the olive oil in a deep, heavy frying pan, add the shallot and fry over medium-high heat for about 1 minute.

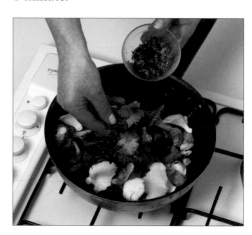

3 Add the garlic, mushrooms and fresh herbs to the pan and sauté for about 5 minutes. Season to taste. Split open the rolls by cutting a cross in the top, then divide the mushrooms among them. Garnish with sprigs of chervil and serve.

VARIATION

For an alternative substantial starch meal, serve the mushrooms with Grilled Polenta or freshly cooked pasta. Served without the rolls, this dish is neutral and would make a tasty appetizer before either a starch or protein main course.

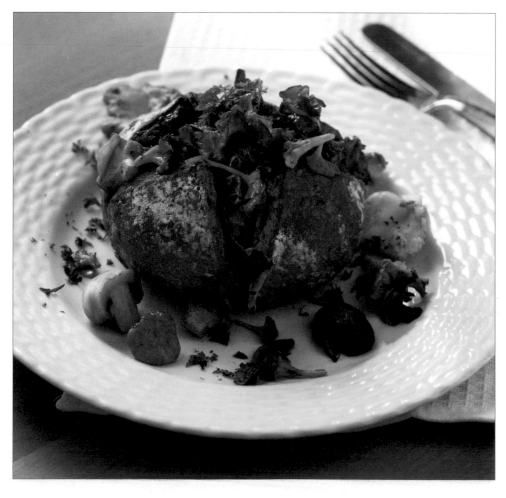

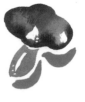

Eggplant and Spinach Terrines (P)

These individual terrines make an elegant first course or accompaniment to either a fish or meat course, cold or hot.

INGREDIENTS

Serves 4
1 eggplant
2 tablespoons extra virgin olive oil
2 zucchini, thinly sliced
leaves from 1 small fresh thyme sprig
4 firm tomatoes, peeled and seeded
4 fresh basil leaves, finely sliced
1 bunch baby spinach leaves
1 garlic clove, crushed
1 tablespoon butter
pinch of freshly grated nutmeg
salt and freshly ground black pepper
½ roasted red bell pepper, skinned and chopped, plus a little balsamic vinegar, to serve

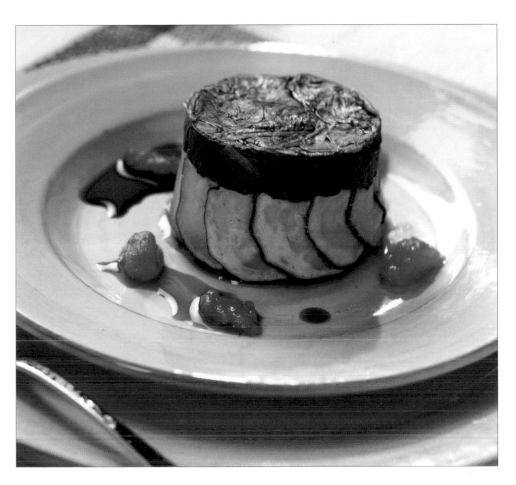

1 Preheat the oven to 375°F and seal four 2½-inch diameter metal muffin rings at one end with plastic wrap.

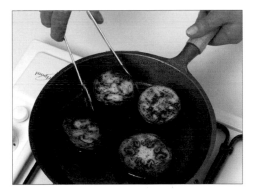

2 Slice the eggplant into four equal-sized rounds. Heat half the oil in a frying pan and fry the eggplant on both sides until brown. Place the eggplant slices on a baking sheet and cook for 10 minutes. Transfer to a plate lined with paper towels.

3 Heat half the remaining oil in the same pan and fry the zucchini for 2 minutes, then drain on the paper towels. Season with salt and pepper and sprinkle with thyme leaves.

4 Place the tomatoes, basil and the rest of the oil in a heavy frying pan and cook for 5–8 minutes. Cook the spinach, garlic and butter in a saucepan, letting all the water evaporate. Drain and add the nutmeg and season with salt and pepper.

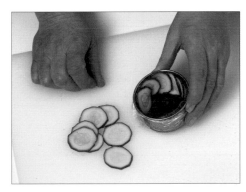

5 Line the base and about ½ inch of the sides of the muffin rings with the spinach leaves, making sure the leaves overlap, leaving no gaps. Place the zucchini around the edges of each ring, overlapping slightly.

6 Divide the tomato mixture equally among the rings, pressing down well. Place the eggplant slices on the top, trimming the edges to fit.

7 Seal the top with plastic wrap and pierce the base to let any liquid escape. Chill overnight. Remove carefully from the rings and serve with diced roasted peppers, drizzled with balsamic vinegar.

COOK'S TIP

Double or triple the quantities in this recipe to make a vegetarian main course and serve with a crisp green salad and a sharp lemon and oil dressing.

Mixed Green Leaf and Herb Salad (N)

Serve this salad as a side dish, or turn it into a main course by using one of the variations, right.

Ingredients

Serves 4

½ cup mixed fresh herbs, such as chervil, tarragon (use sparingly), dill, basil, marjoram (use sparingly), flat-leaf parsley, mint, sorrel, fennel and cilantro

12 ounces mixed salad leaves, such as arugula, radicchio, chicory, watercress, curly endive, baby spinach, nasturtium (and the flowers) and dandelion

For the dressing

¼ cup extra virgin olive oil
1 tablespoon sherry vinegar
salt and freshly ground black pepper

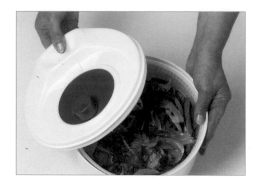

1 Wash and dry the herbs and salad leaves using a salad spinner or place them between two clean, dry dish towels and carefully pat dry.

2 Combine the oil and vinegar and season well.

3 Place the salad and herbs in a large bowl, add the dressing and mix well using your hands to toss the leaves. The dressing should be added just before serving.

Variations

For a protein main course, add one of the following:
• Freshly broiled salmon or tuna or cooked peeled shrimp, either cold or broiled, and lightly dusted with chili powder.
• Fat slices of mozzarella cheese with pitted black olives and a few green capers.
• Slivers of Pecorino cheese with bite-size pieces of crisp pear.

For a starch main course, add one of the following:
• Tiny new potatoes, unpeeled, crumbled hard-cooked egg yolks, bean sprouts.
• Baby fava beans, sliced artichoke hearts and garlic croutons.
• Cooked chickpeas, asparagus tips and pitted green olives stuffed with peppers.

Feta and Apple Salad (P)

Ingredients

Serves 4

3 tablespoons olive oil
juice of 1 lime
½ teaspoon English mustard powder
1 red apple
1 green apple
2 cups arugula
1 cup bean sprouts
2 scallions, finely chopped
1 teaspoon chopped fresh basil
2 teaspoons snipped fresh chives
2 teaspoons chopped fresh chervil
1 teaspoon chopped fresh tarragon
2 tablespoons chopped walnuts
6 ounces feta cheese
salt and freshly ground black pepper

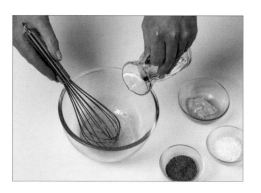

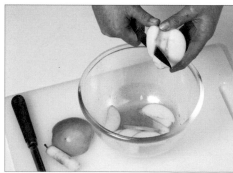

1 Pour the olive oil and lime juice into a large bowl and mix with the mustard, salt and black pepper.

Variation

As an alternative to feta, which is rather salty, you could use a milder but still crumbly cheese such as Caerphilly.

2 Core the apples, slice into thin shavings and mix with the dressing in the bowl. Add the arugula, bean sprouts, scallions, herbs and walnuts and mix well.

3 Serve in one large serving bowl or in four individual bowls with the feta cheese crumbled on top.

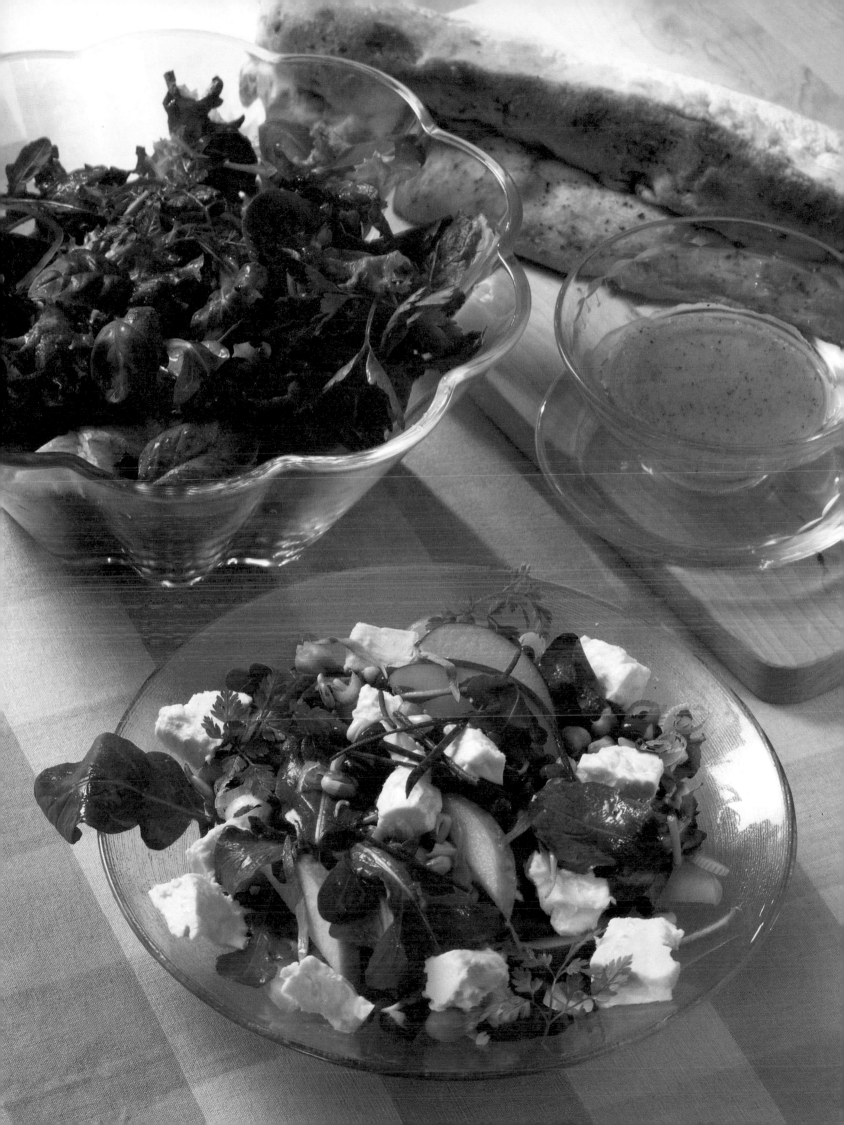

Asian Salad (N)

This fragrantly flavored salad combines with either starch or protein meals. The dressing may be used for any combination of raw vegetables and salad greens.

INGREDIENTS

Serves 4
2 cups bean sprouts
1 cucumber
2 carrots
1 small daikon radish
1 small red onion, thinly sliced
1-inch piece fresh ginger, peeled and
    cut into thin matchsticks
1 small red chili, seeded and
    thinly sliced
handful of fresh cilantro leaves or fresh
    mint leaves

For the Asian dressing
1 tablespoon rice vinegar
1 tablespoon light soy sauce
1 tablespoon *nam pla* (Thai fish sauce)
1 garlic clove, finely chopped
1 tablespoon sesame oil
3 tablespoons peanut oil
2 tablespoons sesame seeds,
    lightly toasted

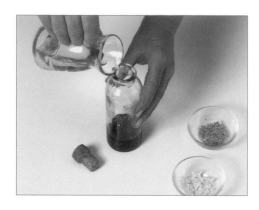

1 First make the dressing. Place all the dressing ingredients in a bottle or an airtight jar and shake well.

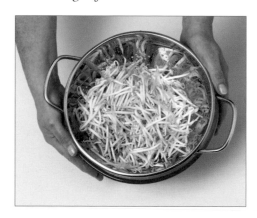

2 Wash the bean sprouts and drain thoroughly in a colander.

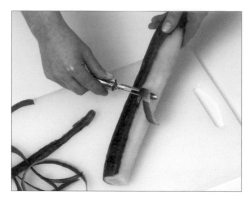

3 Peel the cucumber, cut it in half lengthwise and carefully scoop out the seeds. Peel the cucumber flesh into long ribbon strips using a potato peeler.

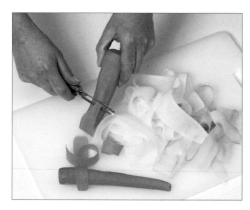

4 Peel the carrots and radish into long strips in the same way as the cucumber.

5 Place the carrots, radish and cucumber in a large shallow serving dish, add the onion, ginger, chili and cilantro and toss to mix. Pour the dressing on just before serving.

—— COOK'S TIP ——

The dressing may be made in advance and will keep well for a couple of days if stored in the refrigerator or a cool place.

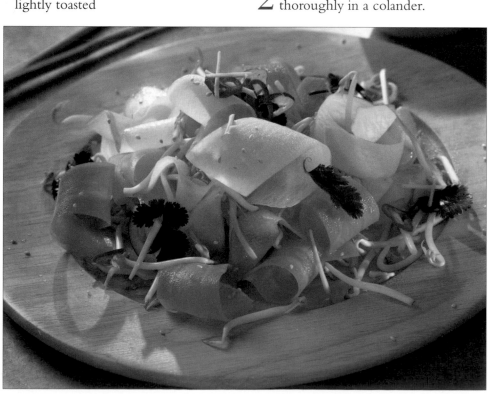

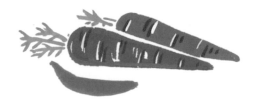

Fennel and Herb Coleslaw (N)

This neutral salad may be easily adapted into a protein meal with the addition of generous chunks of feta, or any other crumbly and salty cheese, and slices of crisp red apples.

INGREDIENTS

Serves 4
1 bulb fennel
2 scallions
1 small white cabbage
2 stalks celery
4 small carrots
¼ cup golden raisins
½ teaspoon caraway seeds (optional)
1 tablespoon chopped fresh parsley
3 tablespoons extra virgin olive oil
1 teaspoon lemon juice
shreds of scallions, to garnish

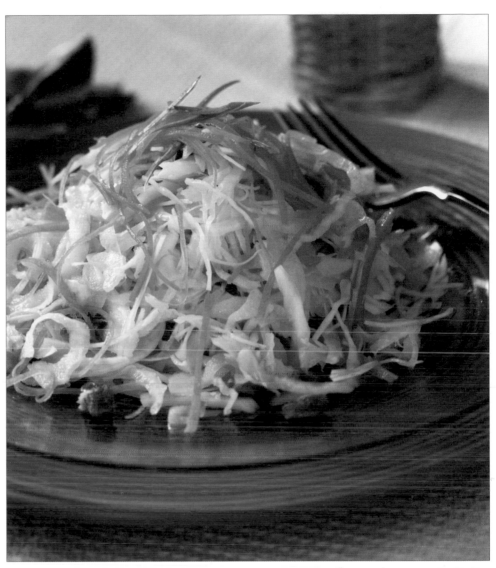

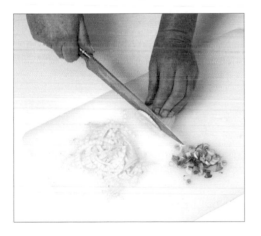

1 Using a sharp knife, cut the fennel and scallions into thin slices.

VARIATION

Use sour cream instead of olive oil for a creamier dressing.

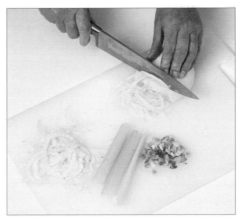

2 Slice the cabbage and celery finely and cut the carrots into fine strips. Place in a serving bowl with the other vegetables. Add the raisins and caraway seeds, if using, and toss lightly to mix.

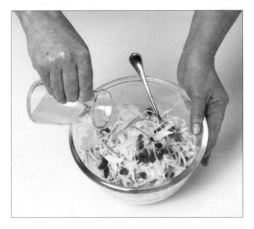

3 Stir in the chopped parsley, olive oil and lemon juice and mix all the ingredients very thoroughly. Cover and chill for 3 hours to let the flavors mingle, and then serve, garnished with scallion shreds.

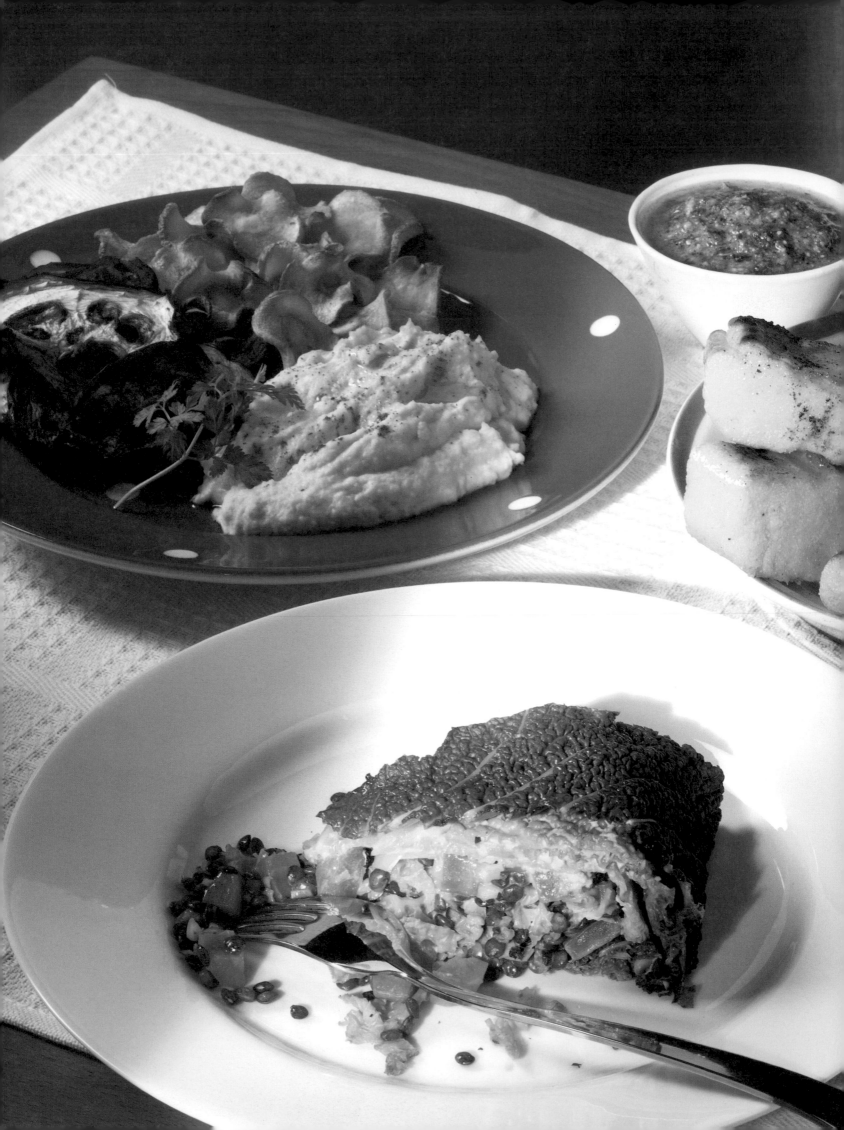

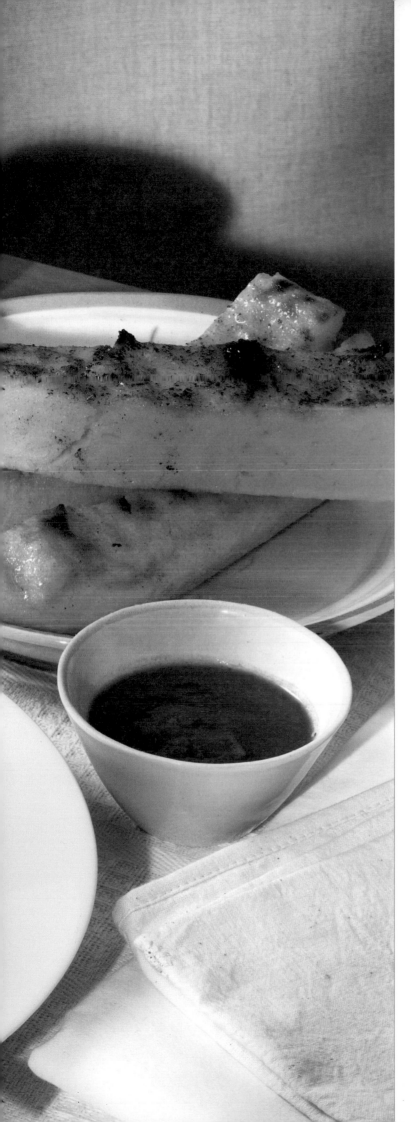

GRAINS, BEANS AND RICE

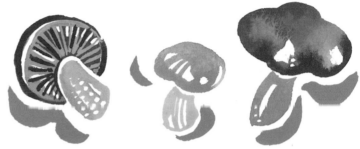

If you have always thought of grains and beans as dull and stodgy you will be pleasantly surprised by the flavor and texture of Cracked Wheat Salad and Bean Feast with its sharp and pungent Tomato and Avocado Salsa. Freshly made Hummus is much more wholesome and crunchy when made with sprouted chickpeas and is irresistible with lots of piping hot Vegetable Chips. While all these recipes are indicated as starch dishes, beans and legumes do contain some protein, which is important for vegetarians.

Falafel with Tahini Dressing (S)

Falafel or chickpea rissoles are a popular Middle Eastern snack. Serve them with a green leaf salad and pita bread.

INGREDIENTS

Serves 4

1½ cups dried chickpeas, soaked overnight
1 large onion, finely chopped
4 scallions, finely chopped
3 tablespoons chopped fresh cilantro
3 tablespoons chopped fresh parsley
1 teaspoon ground coriander
1 teaspoon ground fennel seeds
1 teaspoon ground cumin
½ teaspoon baking powder
2 garlic cloves, crushed
sunflower oil, for frying
salt and freshly ground black pepper
pinch of paprika and chopped fresh cilantro, to garnish

For the dressing
3 tablespoons tahini

1 Drain the chickpeas and cook in plenty of boiling water for 1–1½ hours, until tender.

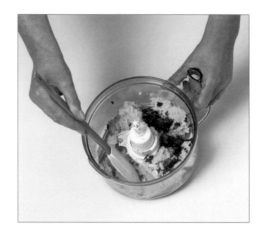

2 Drain the chickpeas and process in a blender or food processor until they form a smooth paste. Add the onion and scallions, cilantro and parsley, process again for a few seconds and then add the ground spices, baking powder and crushed garlic. Season with salt and pepper.

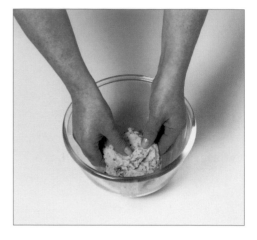

3 Transfer the mixture to a bowl and knead with your hands until pliable, then let it rest in the refrigerator for at least 30 minutes.

4 Meanwhile, make the dressing. Place the tahini in a bowl and gradually add ½ cup water, to make a smooth paste, the consistency of cream. Season with salt and pepper and spoon into a serving bowl. Chill until ready to serve.

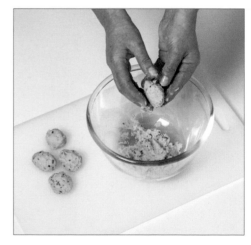

5 Take walnut-size pieces of the mixture and form into small balls about 1½ inches across. Heat a little oil in a frying pan and fry the falafel, three or four at a time, for about 3 minutes on each side, until golden brown. Drain on paper towels and keep warm. Repeat with the remaining falafels. Arrange on a serving plate, dust with paprika and garnish with fresh cilantro. Serve with the tahini dressing.

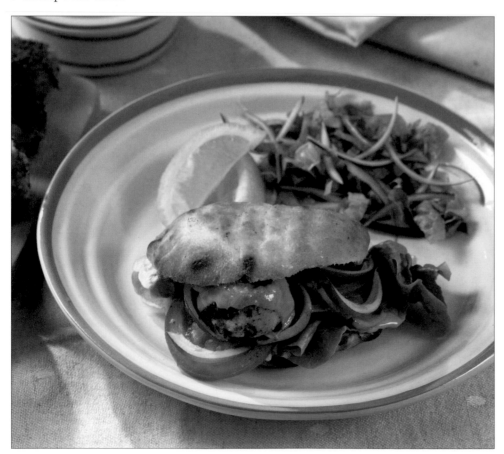

Hummus with Baked Vegetable Chips (S)

This classic Middle Eastern appetizer is ideally made using sprouted chickpeas, which are available at health food stores and most good supermarkets. Canned chickpeas are a useful standby and can be used instead of the sprouted chickpeas—rinse them thoroughly before using.

INGREDIENTS

Serves 4
1 pound sprouted chickpeas or 1 can (14 ounces) chickpeas
2 garlic cloves, crushed
¼ cup tahini
¼ cup extra virgin olive oil
2 tablespoons lemon juice
salt
small pinch of paprika and sprigs of flat-leaf parsley or chervil, to garnish

For the vegetable chips
2 large eggplants
4 large parsnips
1 teaspoon extra virgin olive oil

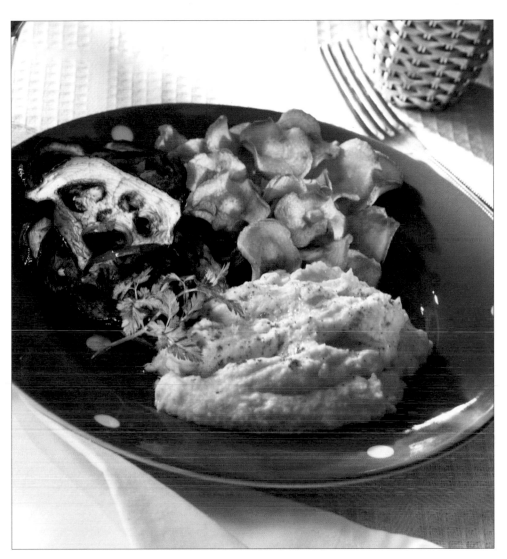

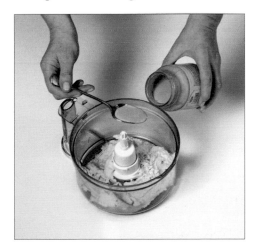

1 Blend the chickpeas in a food processor until completely smooth. Add the garlic, tahini and a little salt.

—— COOK'S TIP ——

To make a rich sauce for steamed vegetables, just add a little more water.

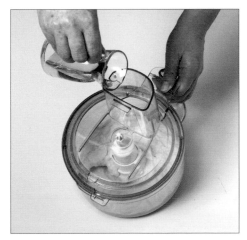

2 With the machine running, slowly pour in the olive oil to make a thick, smooth sauce and then add the lemon juice. If the mixture is too thick, add a little water. Transfer to a serving bowl and set aside.

3 Preheat the oven to 250°F. Slice the eggplants and parsnips into very thin rounds. Brush both sides of the vegetable slices with olive oil and sprinkle with a little salt.

4 Place on oven racks and bake for 30 minutes, until golden brown and crisp. The vegetables may take longer, so continue cooking, checking every 10 minutes.

5 Serve the vegetable chips with the hummus, garnished with a light dusting of paprika and sprigs of fresh parsley or chervil.

Cracked Wheat Salad with Walnuts and Herbs (S)

INGREDIENTS

Serves 4

1 generous cup cracked wheat
1½ cups vegetable stock
1 cinnamon stick
generous pinch of ground cumin
pinch of cayenne pepper
pinch of ground cloves
1 teaspoon salt, finely ground
10 snow peas, trimmed
1 red and 1 yellow bell pepper, roasted,
   skinned, seeded and diced
2 plum tomatoes, peeled, seeded
   and diced
2 shallots, finely sliced
5 black olives, pitted and cut
   into quarters
2 tablespoons each shredded fresh basil,
   mint and parsley
2 tablespoons roughly chopped walnuts
2 tablespoons balsamic vinegar
½ cup extra virgin olive oil
freshly ground black pepper
onion rings, to garnish

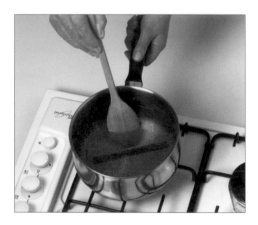

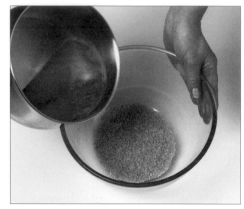

1 Place the cracked wheat in a large bowl. Pour the stock into a saucepan and bring to a boil with the spices and salt.

2 Cook for 1 minute, then pour the stock over the cracked wheat and let stand for 30 minutes.

— COOK'S TIP —

To roast the peppers, cut in half and place skin side up on a baking tray. Place in an oven preheated to 425°F and roast for about 20 minutes, until the skins are charred. Place the peppers in a plastic bag, knot the end and let sit for 10 minutes. Then the skin can be simply pulled off.

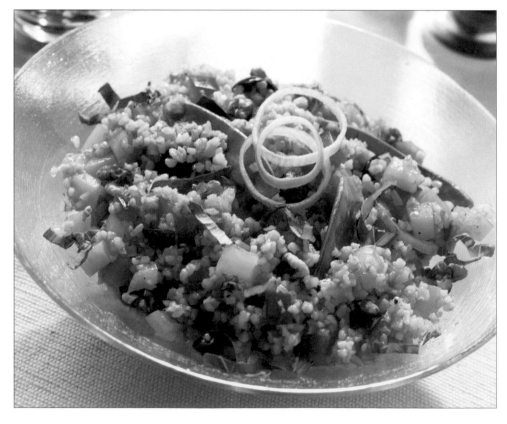

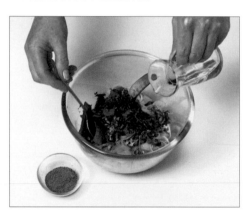

3 In another bowl, combine the snow peas, peppers, tomatoes, shallots, olives, herbs and walnuts. Add the vinegar, olive oil and a little black pepper and stir thoroughly to mix.

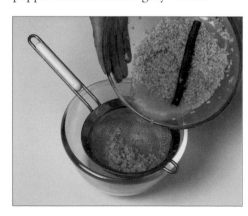

4 Strain the cracked wheat and discard the cinnamon stick. Place in a serving bowl, stir in the fresh vegetable mixture and serve, garnished with onion rings.

Savoy Cabbage and Vegetable Pie (S)

Before cooking the lentils, spread them out on a plate to make sure there are no pieces of grit, which can seriously damage your teeth! Serve this pie with baked potatoes, or new potatoes steamed in their skins.

INGREDIENTS

Serves 4

1 small savoy cabbage, outer leaves removed
3 tablespoons olive oil
1 shallot, finely chopped
1 garlic clove, finely chopped
1 carrot, cut into small dice
1 leek, white part only, cut into thin slices
1 celery stalk, cut into small dice
1 tablespoon pine nuts
1 bay leaf
½ cup Puy lentils
2¼ cups vegetable stock
5 tablespoons heavy cream
3 egg yolks
salt and freshly ground black pepper

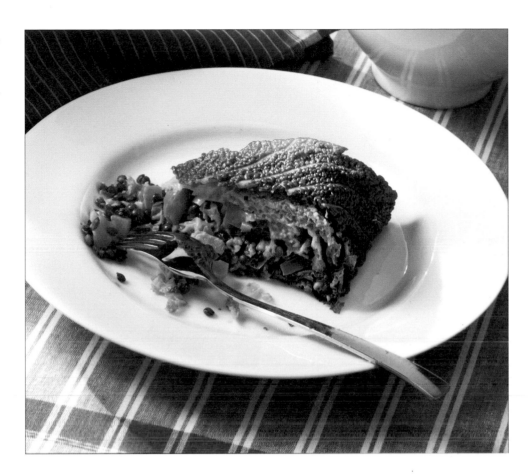

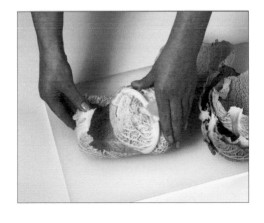

1 Pull away ten large undamaged cabbage leaves and blanch them in a saucepan of boiling water for 1 minute. Plunge into a bowl of ice-cold water for 30 seconds and drain immediately.

2 Cut the remaining cabbage into quarters, cut out and discard the stalk and slice very thinly.

3 Heat the oil in a heavy saucepan and fry the shallot for 3 minutes, until softened. Add the garlic, sliced cabbage, carrot, leek, celery, pine nuts and bay leaf and cook for another 3 minutes, stirring frequently.

4 Add the lentils and vegetable stock to the pan, cover and simmer for about 30 minutes, until the lentils are tender and the liquid has evaporated. Let cool. Preheat the oven to 400°F.

5 Line a 6-inch tart pan with seven of the cabbage leaves and season with salt and pepper.

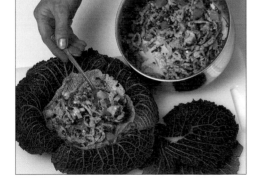

6 Blend the cream with the egg yolks and stir into the lentil mixture. Season to taste, then spoon the mixture into the cabbage ring and cover with the remaining leaves. Cover with foil and cook for 40 minutes. Once the pie is cooked, let it stand, still covered with foil, for 10 minutes before slicing into thick wedges to serve.

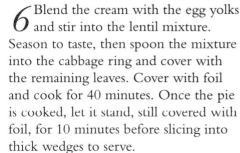

Wild Rice and Grain Pilaf with Mushrooms (S)

INGREDIENTS

Serves 4
¼ cup wheat berries
2 tablespoons butter
1 shallot, finely chopped
¼ cup wild rice
2½ cups vegetable stock
1 bay leaf
¼ cup brown basmati rice
1½ cups shiitake mushrooms
1½ cups brown-cap mushrooms
2 tablespoons olive oil
4 scallions, thinly sliced
¼ cup hazelnuts, roughly chopped
salt and freshly ground black pepper

1 Rinse the wheat berries, cover with 4 cups boiling water and let soak for at least 2 hours or overnight. Drain.

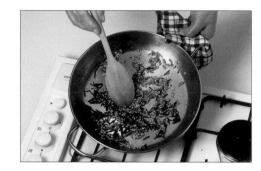

2 Melt the butter in a heavy frying pan and fry the shallot for 3 minutes. Add the wheat berries and wild rice, stir well to coat the grains, and then add the stock, bay leaf and ½ teaspoon salt. Bring to a boil, then lower the heat, cover and simmer for 30 minutes.

3 Stir in the brown basmati rice and simmer for another 20 minutes. Remove from the heat and let stand for 5 minutes.

4 Quarter the shiitake mushrooms and remove and discard the stems. Quarter the brown-cap mushrooms. Heat the olive oil in another frying pan and fry the mushrooms for 3 minutes, stirring well. Add the scallions and hazelnuts and cook for another 1 minute.

5 Strain any liquid from the rice and then stir in the mushrooms. Season with salt and pepper to taste and serve.

Broiled Polenta (S)

Polenta is coarse yellow corn meal and is one of the staples of northern Italy where it often replaces bread. A couple of slices of broiled polenta with Stargazer Vegetable Soup and a hearty salad make a well-balanced and satisfying lunch. It is also delicious with Mixed Mushroom Sandwiches.

INGREDIENTS
Serves 4
3¾ cups water
1¼ cups polenta
2 tablespoons butter
1 teaspoon extra virgin olive oil
salt and freshly ground black pepper

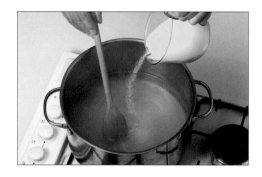

1 Boil the water in a large heavy saucepan and add 1 teaspoon salt. Reduce the heat until the water is just simmering and slowly pour in the polenta, stirring vigorously, until completely blended.

2 Reduce the heat, and cook for 40 minutes, stirring every 5 minutes with a wooden spoon. The polenta is cooked when it is very thick and falls away from the sides of the pan.

3 Stir in the butter and seasoning and transfer to a flat baking sheet. Spread out until about 1 inch thick and set aside until completely cold.

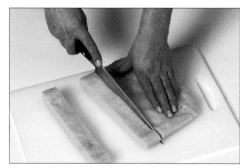

4 Cut the polenta into wedges or slices and brush each piece lightly with olive oil. Place under a hot broiler until each slice is crisp and brown on both sides. Serve hot.

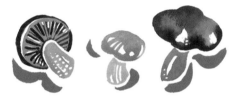

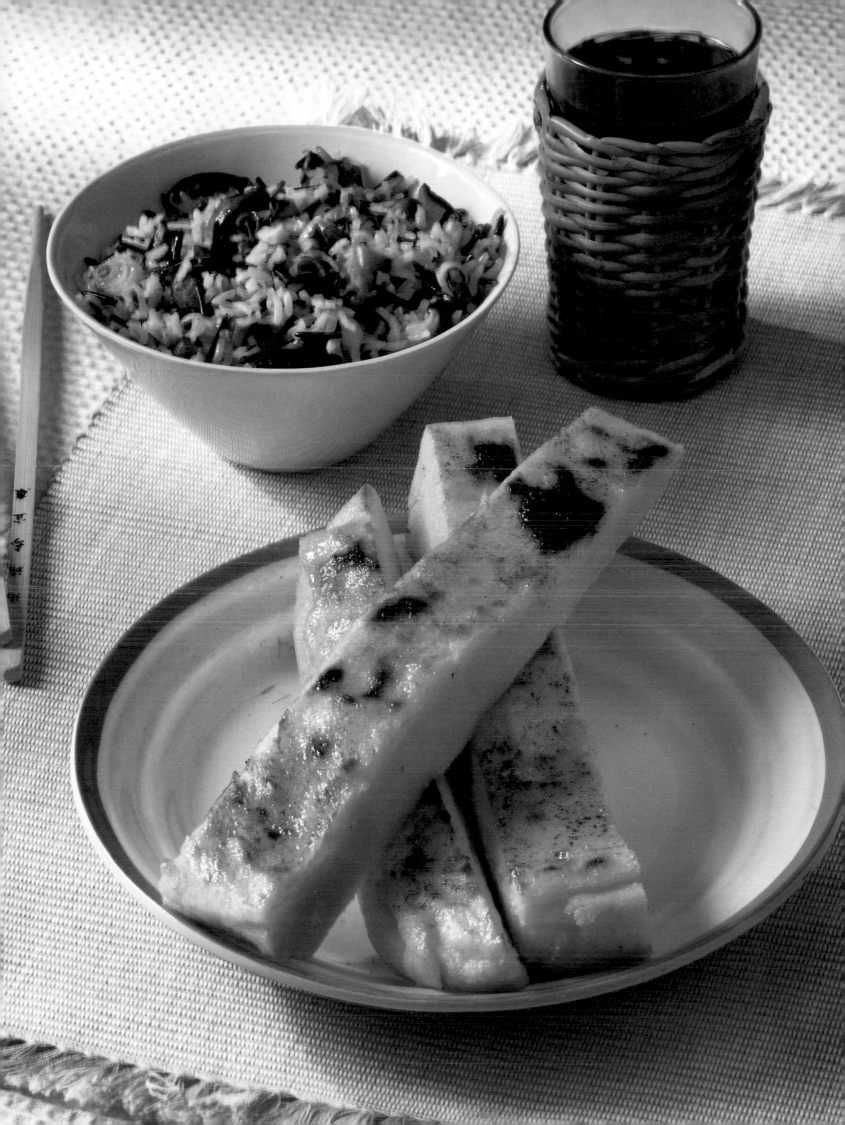

Lentil Risotto with Vegetables (S)

INGREDIENTS

Serves 4

3 tablespoons sunflower oil
1 large onion, thinly sliced
2 garlic cloves, crushed
1 large carrot, cut into matchsticks
1 generous cup brown basmati rice,
   washed and drained
½ cup green or brown lentils, soaked
   overnight and drained
1 teaspoon ground cumin
1 teaspoon ground cinnamon
20 black cardamom seeds
6 cloves
2½ cups vegetable stock
2 bay leaves
2 celery stalks
1 large avocado
3 plum tomatoes
salt and freshly ground black pepper
green salad, to serve

1 Heat the oil in a heavy pan and fry the onion, garlic and carrot for 5–6 minutes, until the onion is transparent and the carrot is slightly softened.

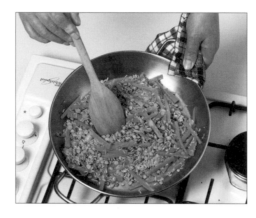

2 Add the drained rice and lentils together with the cumin, cinnamon, cardamom seeds and cloves and continue frying over low heat for another 5 minutes, stirring well to prevent sticking.

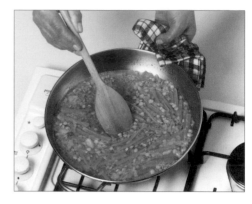

3 Add the vegetable stock and bay leaves and bring to a boil, then cover the pan and simmer very gently for another 15 minutes or until the liquid has been absorbed and the rice and lentils are tender. Taste and adjust the seasoning.

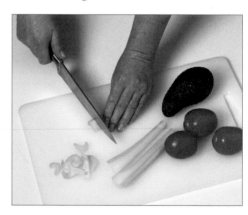

4 Meanwhile, chop the celery into half-rounds and dice the avocado and tomatoes.

5 Add the fresh ingredients to the rice and lentils and stir to mix. Spoon into a large serving bowl and serve immediately with a green salad.

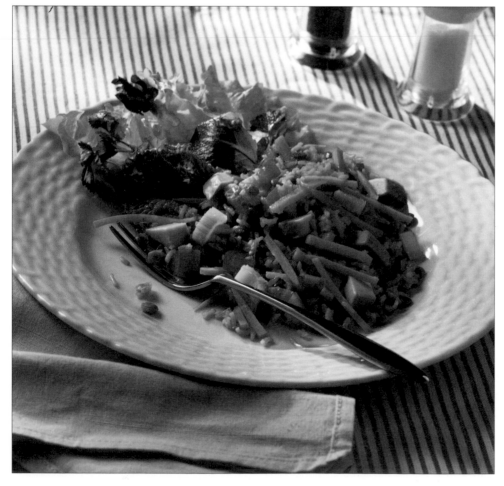

Bean Feast with Tomato and Avocado Salsa (S)

This is a super-quick recipe using canned beans, although it could be made with dried beans, which would need to be soaked overnight and then cooked for 1–1¹/₂ hours until tender.

INGREDIENTS

Serves 4

1 can (14 ounces) red kidney beans
1 can (14 ounces) flageolet beans
1 can (14 ounces) borlotti beans
1 tablespoon olive oil
1 small onion, finely chopped
3 garlic cloves, finely chopped
1 red ancho chili, seeded and
    finely chopped
1 red bell pepper, seeded and
    coarsely chopped
2 bay leaves
2 teaspoons chopped fresh oregano
2 teaspoons ground cumin
1 teaspoon ground coriander
¹/₂ teaspoon ground cloves
1 tablespoon dark brown sugar
1¹/₄ cups vegetable stock
salt and freshly ground black pepper
sprigs of fresh cilantro, to garnish

For the salsa
1 ripe but firm avocado
3 tablespoons fresh lime juice
1 small red onion
1 small hot green chili
3 ripe plum tomatoes
3 tablespoons chopped fresh cilantro

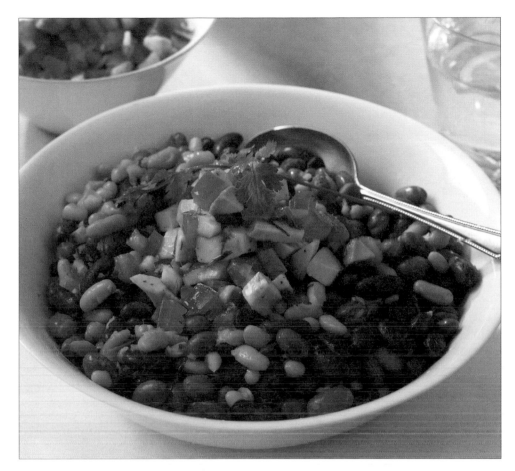

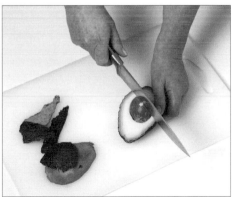

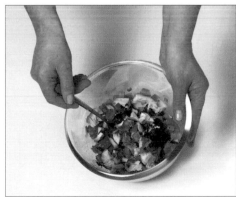

1 Drain the beans in a colander and rinse thoroughly. Heat the oil in a heavy saucepan and fry the onion for 3 minutes, until soft and transparent. Add the garlic, chili, red pepper, herbs and spices.

2 Stir well and cook for another 3 minutes, then add the sugar, beans and stock and cook for 8 minutes. Season with salt and pepper.

3 To make the salsa, peel the avocado, cut it in half around the pit, then remove the pit using a large sharp knife. Cut the flesh into ¹/₂-inch dice. Place in a mixing bowl with the lime juice and stir to mix.

4 Roughly chop the onion and finely slice the chili, discarding the seeds. Plunge the tomatoes into boiling water, let sit for 1 minute and then peel away the skin. Chop the tomatoes into rough pieces and discard the seeds.

5 Add the onion, chili, tomatoes and cilantro to the avocado. Season with black pepper and stir to mix.

6 Spoon the beans into a warmed serving dish or into four serving bowls. Serve with the tomato and avocado salsa and garnish with sprigs of fresh cilantro.

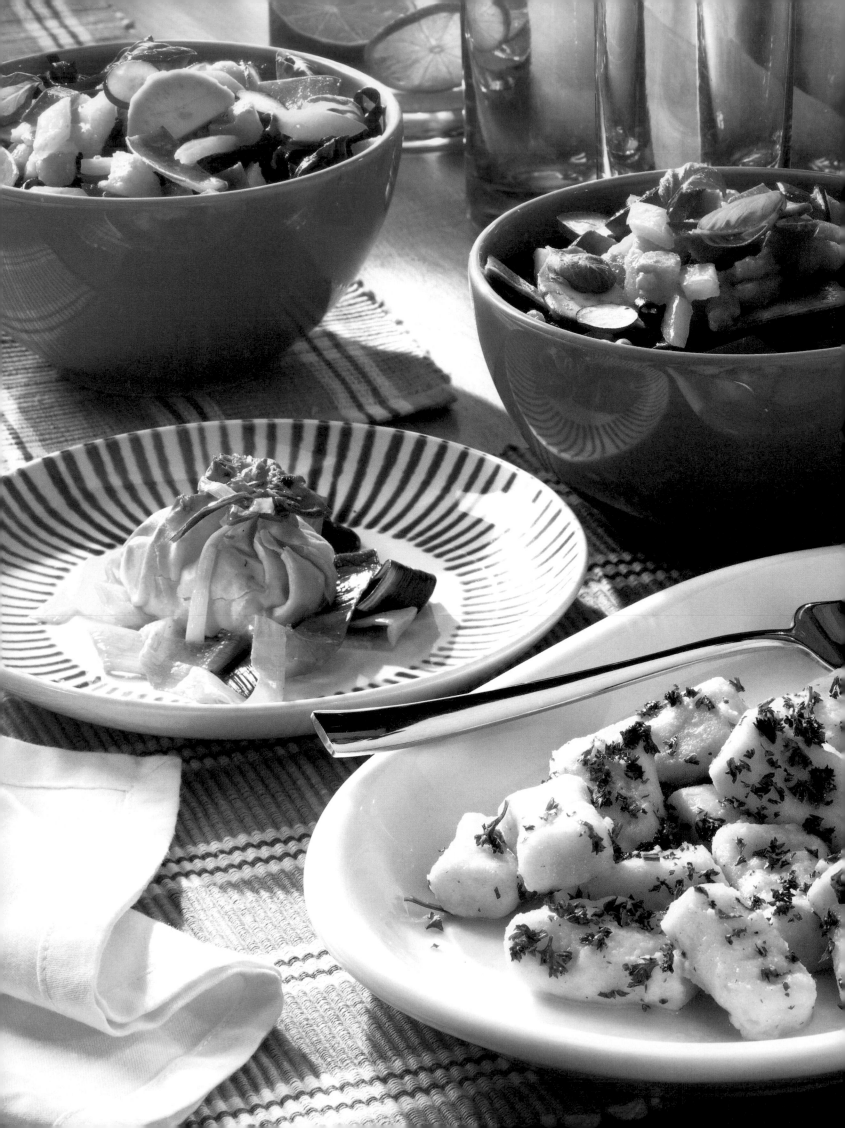

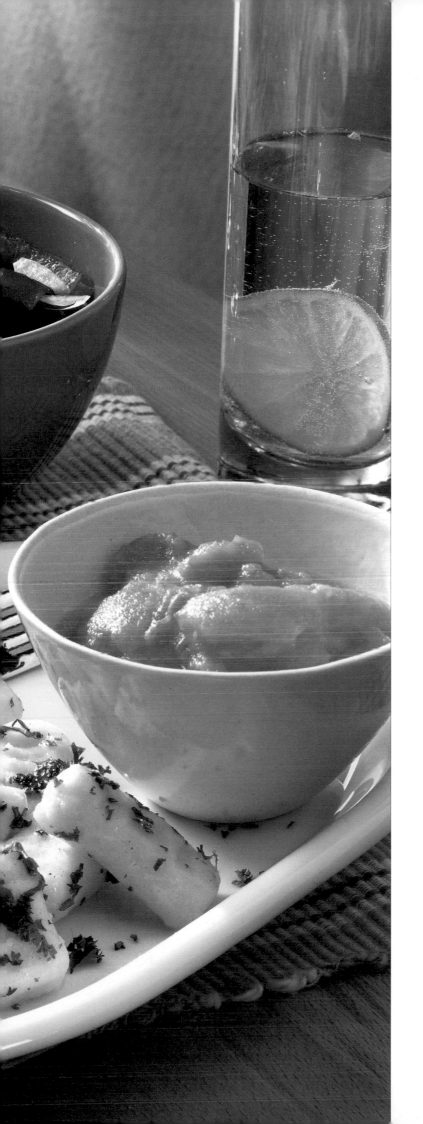

PASTA AND PASTRY

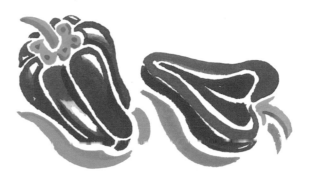

Pasta or gnocchi makes a filling starch meal especially when combined with one of the different and original sauces included here. The sauces can also be served with brown rice or spooned onto split baked potatoes or lightly steamed vegetables. While making pastry with whole-wheat flour is recommended, it does no harm to your diet to occasionally use the ready-made, light and super-thin filo pastry, especially when it is filled with plenty of tasty Mediterranean vegetables or used to encase a subtle combination of cream cheese, leeks and fresh herbs.

Chinese Primavera (S)

INGREDIENTS

Serves 4

12 ounces capellini pasta (egg-free)
½ teaspoon salt
1 tablespoon peanut oil
1 red bell pepper, seeded
1 yellow bell pepper, seeded
1 cup snow peas
10 button mushrooms
3 scallions
2 tablespoons cornstarch
1 tablespoon olive oil
3 garlic cloves, finely chopped
¾ cup vegetable stock
3 tablespoons dry sherry
2 tablespoons sesame oil
1 tablespoon light soy sauce
1 teaspoon chili sauce
1 tablespoon oyster sauce
½ teaspoon superfine sugar
½ teaspoon Szechuan peppercorns,
    crushed
rind of 1 orange, cut into thin shreds,
    to garnish

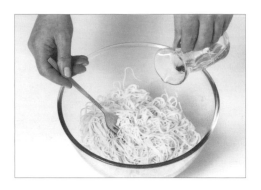

1 Place the pasta in a large pot of boiling water with the salt, and cook for 3 minutes. Drain in a colander and then transfer to a large bowl and stir in the peanut oil.

— COOK'S TIP —

Capellini, vermicelli and angel hair pasta cook very quickly and are ideal for quick meals. Serve with slices of fresh tomato sprinkled with chopped basil leaves and a little extra virgin olive oil.

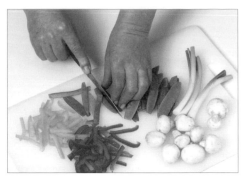

2 Cut the peppers into matchsticks, halve the snow peas, thinly slice the mushrooms and shred the scallions. Stir them into the pasta.

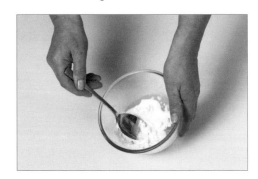

3 Blend the cornstarch with 2 tablespoons water in a bowl.

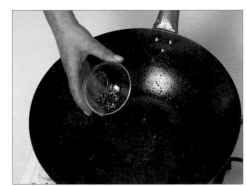

4 Heat the olive oil in a wok and stir-fry the garlic for 20 seconds. Add the vegetable stock, sherry, sesame oil, soy, chili and oyster sauces, sugar and peppercorns. Bring to a boil and pour in the cornstarch mixture, stirring constantly.

5 Add the pasta and vegetables and heat through for 2 minutes. Serve immediately, garnished with orange rind.

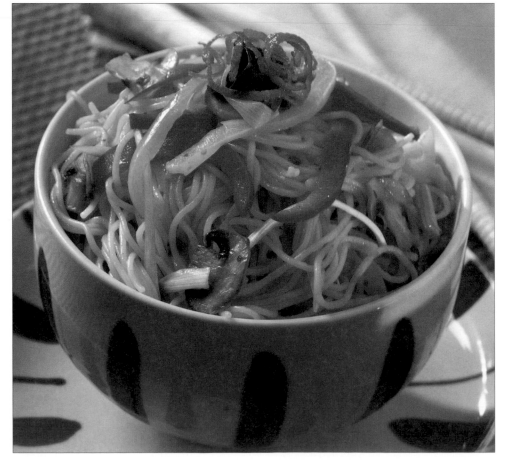

Black Pasta with Raw Vegetables (S)

Black pasta derives its dramatic color from the addition of squid ink. Alternatively you could use Japanese soba or buckwheat noodles, which have a nutty flavor and texture.

INGREDIENTS

Serves 4

3 garlic cloves, crushed
2 tablespoons white tarragon vinegar
1 teaspoon Dijon mustard
6 tablespoons extra virgin olive oil
1 teaspoon finely chopped fresh thyme
1 yellow bell pepper, seeded
1 red bell pepper, seeded
1½ cups snow peas, trimmed
6 radishes
4 ripe plum tomatoes, peeled
 and seeded
1 avocado
10 ounces black pasta (egg-free)
salt and freshly ground black pepper
6 fresh basil leaves, to garnish

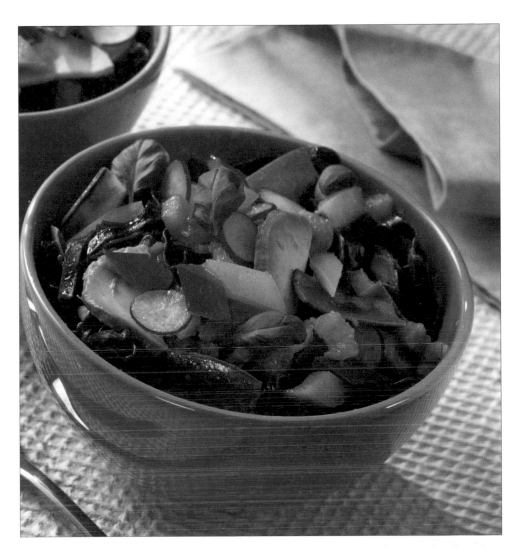

1 In a large bowl, combine the garlic, vinegar, mustard, olive oil and chopped thyme. Season to taste with salt and pepper.

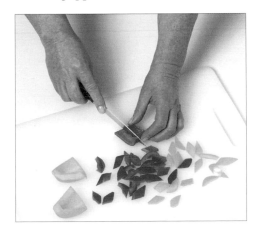

2 Cut the peppers into diamond shapes, halve the snow peas and slice the radishes.

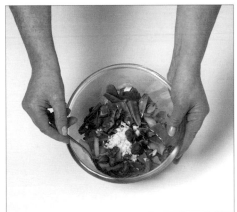

3 Dice the tomatoes. Peel, pit and slice the avocado. Place all the vegetables in a bowl and add the dressing, stirring thoroughly to mix.

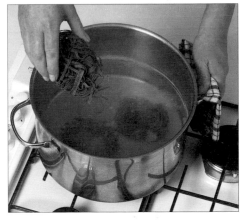

4 Cook the pasta in plenty of slightly salted boiling water until *al dente*. The cooking time will vary depending on the type of pasta. Drain and transfer to a large shallow serving dish. Cover with the vegetables and serve immediately, garnished with basil.

Zucchini and Dill Tart (S)

It is worth making your own pastry for this tart. Although store-bought pastry is a useful standby, it never tastes quite as good as homemade.

INGREDIENTS

Serves 4
1 cup whole-wheat flour
1 cup self-rising flour
8 tablespoons (1 stick) unsalted butter, chilled and diced
5 tablespoons ice-cold water
pinch salt

For the filling
1 tablespoon sunflower oil
3 zucchini, thinly sliced
2 egg yolks
$^2/_3$ cup heavy cream
1 garlic clove, crushed
1 tablespoon finely chopped fresh dill
salt and freshly ground black pepper

1 Sift the flours into a bowl, returning any of the wheat bran into the bowl, then place in a food processor. Add the salt and butter and process using the pulse button until the mixture resembles fine bread crumbs.

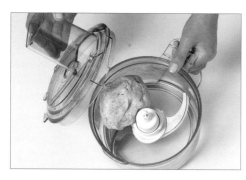

2 Gradually add the water until the mixture forms a dough. Do not overprocess. Rest the pastry by wrapping it in plastic wrap and placing in the refrigerator for 30 minutes.

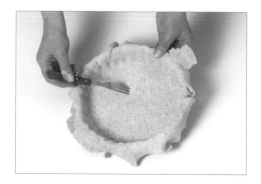

3 Preheat the oven to 400°F and grease an 8-inch tart pan. Roll out the pastry and ease into the pan. Prick the base with a fork and bake "blind" for 10–15 minutes, until golden brown.

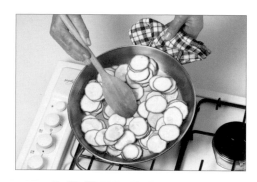

4 Meanwhile, heat the oil in a frying pan and sauté the zucchini for 2–3 minutes, until golden brown, turning occasionally. Blend the egg yolks, heavy cream, garlic and dill in a small bowl. Season to taste with salt and pepper.

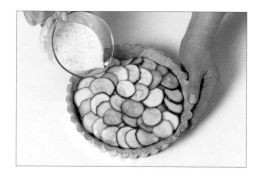

5 Line the pastry shell with layers of zucchini and gently pour in the cream mixture. Return to the oven for 25–30 minutes or until the filling is firm and lightly golden. Cool in the pan and then remove and serve.

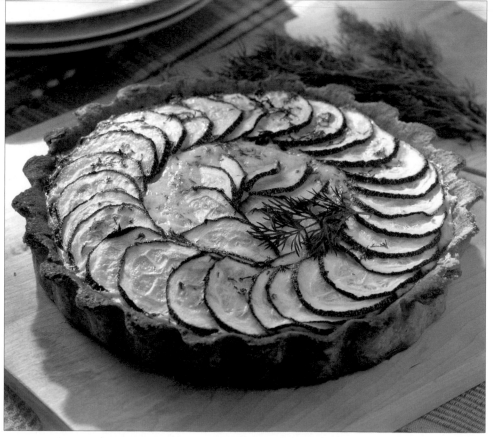

Potato Gnocchi with Fresh Tomato Sauce (S)

Gnocchi make a substantial and tasty alternative to pasta. They are served with a fresh tomato sauce which, because the tomatoes are simply warmed through for a short time, and not cooked, remains neutral.

INGREDIENTS

Serves 4
1½ pounds potatoes, floury type
2 egg yolks
³⁄₄ cup flour
salt
¼ cup finely chopped fresh parsley, to garnish

For the sauce
1 pound plum tomatoes, peeled, seeded and chopped
2 tablespoons melted butter

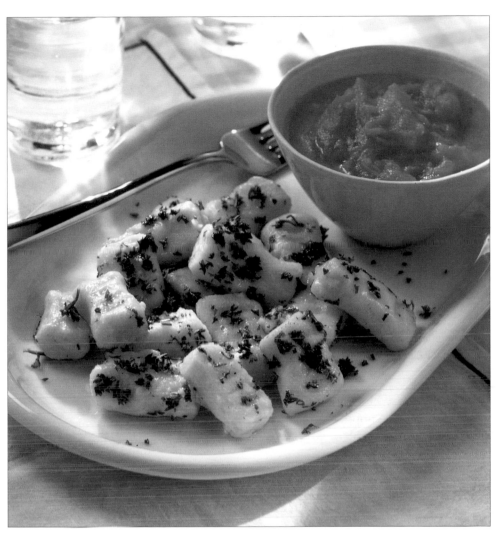

1 Preheat the oven to 400°F. Scrub the potatoes and bake them in their skins for about 1 hour or until the flesh feels soft when pricked with a fork.

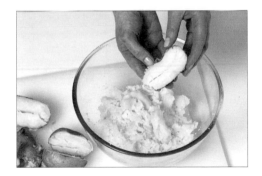

2 Peel the potatoes while still warm, discarding the skins, and mash the flesh well. Add a little salt and stir in the egg yolks.

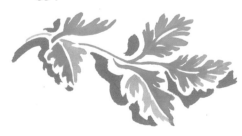

3 Place the potato mixture on a floured surface and knead in the flour to make a smooth elastic dough.

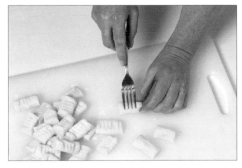

4 Shape the dough into small thumb-shapes by making long rolls and cutting them into segments. Press each gnocchi with the back of a fork to give a ridged effect. Place the gnocchi on a floured surface.

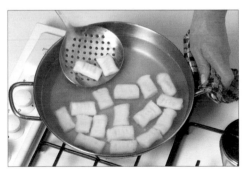

5 Cook the gnocchi in small batches in barely simmering, slightly salted water for about 10 minutes. Remove with a slotted spoon, drain well and keep warm.

6 To make the sauce, cook the tomatoes in the butter in a small pan for 1 minute. Sprinkle the gnocchi with chopped parsley and serve immediately with the sauce.

Filo "Money Bags" with Creamy Leek Filling (S)

Ready-made fresh or frozen filo pastry is widely available at good supermarkets and can be used for both sweet and savory dishes.

INGREDIENTS

Serves 4

8 tablespoons (1 stick) butter
2 cups leeks, trimmed and finely chopped
1 cup cream cheese
1 tablespoon finely chopped fresh dill
1 tablespoon finely chopped fresh parsley
2 scallions, finely chopped
pinch of cayenne pepper
1 garlic clove, finely chopped
½ teaspoon salt
¼ teaspoon freshly ground black pepper
1 egg yolk
9 sheets filo pastry, thawed if frozen
lightly cooked leeks, to serve

1 Preheat the oven to 400°F. Melt 2 tablespoons of the butter in a frying pan and fry the leeks for 4–5 minutes, until soft. Drain off any liquid.

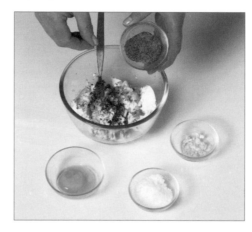

2 Put the cream cheese in a bowl and stir in the dill, parsley, scallions, cayenne pepper, garlic and seasoning. Add the egg yolk and leeks and stir well. Melt the remaining butter.

3 Place one sheet of filo pastry on a board, brush with a little of the melted butter and place another sheet on top. Brush again with butter and top with a third sheet of filo.

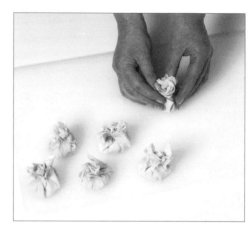

4 Cut the filo into four squares and place 1 rounded tablespoon of the cheese mixture in the center of each square. Gather up the edges into a "bag," twisting the top to seal.

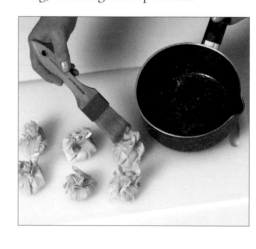

5 Repeat with the other six sheets of filo to make 12 bags. Brush each bag with a little more butter.

6 Place the bags on a greased baking sheet and bake for 20–25 minutes, until golden brown. Serve on a bed of lightly cooked leeks.

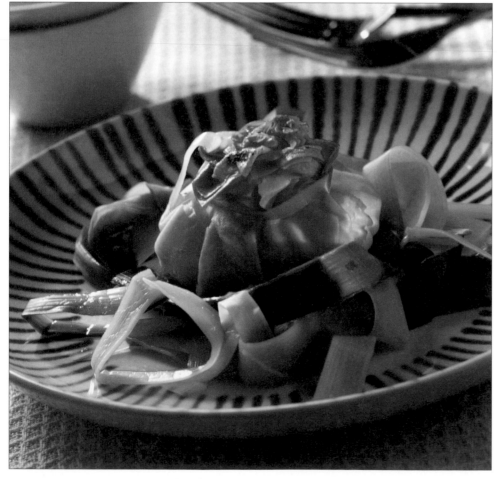

COOK'S TIP

For an attractive effect, tie each bag with a strip of blanched leek before serving.

Filo Baskets with Mediterranean Vegetables (S)

This richly flavored vegetable filling may also be served with freshly cooked pasta or with baked potatoes and sour cream.

INGREDIENTS

Makes about 30
1 small eggplant
8 sheets filo pastry, thawed if frozen
8 tablespoons (1 stick) butter, melted
1 red bell pepper, seeded
1 yellow bell pepper, seeded
1 orange bell pepper, seeded
2 large zucchini, trimmed
1 tablespoon extra virgin olive oil
1 onion, finely chopped
2 garlic cloves, finely chopped
1 fresh thyme sprig
1 teaspoon sugar
1 teaspoon balsamic vinegar
salt and freshly ground black pepper
8 fresh basil leaves, shredded,
    to garnish

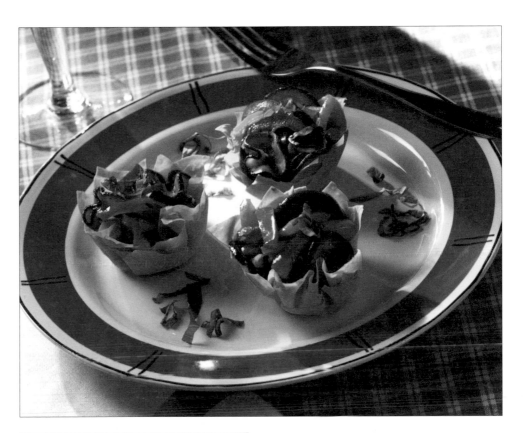

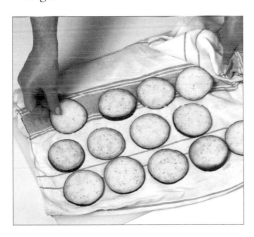

1 Preheat the oven to 350°F. Slice the eggplant into thin rounds, place on a plate or board lined with a clean cloth and sprinkle with salt. Cover with the cloth and place a weighted plate on top. Let sit for about 20 minutes to draw out the juices.

COOK'S TIP

Keep checking the filo baskets while they are baking as they brown very quickly and will become very brittle if overcooked.

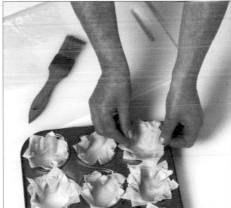

2 Cut two sheets of filo pastry into 15 squares each and brush each square with melted butter. Arrange each square in one cup of a mini muffin pan. Repeat with the remaining filo, to form mini baskets, arranging the squares at angles to create a star effect. Keep the unused filo covered with a damp cloth as you work to prevent it from drying out. Bake for 10 minutes until brown. Cool in the pans.

3 Cut the peppers into strips and slice the zucchini. Rinse the eggplant slices, pat dry and cut in half.

4 Heat the oil in a heavy saucepan and sauté the onion and garlic until soft but not brown. Add the peppers, zucchini, eggplant, thyme and sugar and cook over low heat for 20 minutes, stirring occasionally. Stir in the balsamic vinegar and season with salt and pepper. Remove the sprig of thyme from the pan.

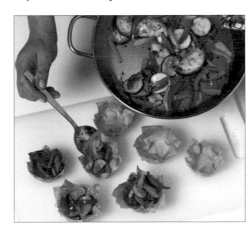

5 Remove the filo baskets from the muffin pans. Divide the vegetable mixture among the baskets and sprinkle each one with shredded basil leaves.

Pasta with Fresh Basil and Parsley Pesto (S)

Choose mixed plain, spinach and tomato pasta for this recipe, or use one of the whole-wheat varieties. The pesto may be made in advance and will keep for a few days in the refrigerator.

INGREDIENTS

Serves 4

14 ounces mixed red, green and natural
pasta shapes (egg-free)

For the pesto

2 garlic cloves, crushed
$^{1}/_{2}$ cup pine nuts
2 cups fresh basil leaves, plus extra to
garnish
$^{1}/_{2}$ cup fresh flat-leaf parsley
$^{2}/_{3}$ cup extra virgin olive oil
salt and freshly ground black pepper

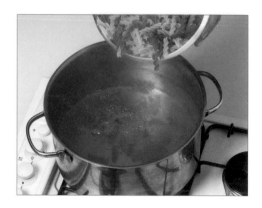

1 Cook the pasta in plenty of lightly salted boiling water until *al dente*. The cooking time will depend on the type of pasta shape you are using.

--- COOK'S TIP ---

To vary the flavor of the pesto, use cilantro instead of parsley.

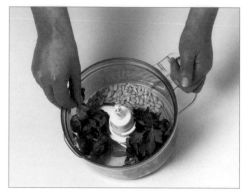

2 Meanwhile, place the garlic, pine nuts, basil, parsley and seasoning in a blender or food processor and process for 30 seconds, while gradually pouring in the oil, to make a thick sauce.

3 Drain the pasta and place on a large warmed serving plate. Pour on the pesto sauce and serve, garnished with extra basil.

Penne with Broccoli and Walnut Sauce (S)

This Italian sauce is truly delicious. It is traditionally served with pasta but can also be spread thickly on slices of fresh or grilled ciabatta bread and served with chunks of celery, tomatoes, cucumber and radishes.

INGREDIENTS

Serves 4

10 ounces dried penne (egg-free)
1 pound fresh broccoli, cut into
equal-size florets

For the sauce

$^{1}/_{2}$ cup walnuts
2 tablespoons fresh brown bread crumbs
$1^{1}/_{2}$ cups fresh parsley
$^{1}/_{2}$ cup extra virgin olive oil
2 tablespoons light cream
salt and freshly ground black pepper

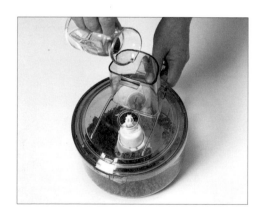

1 First make the sauce. Place the walnuts, bread crumbs and parsley in a blender or food processor and process for 20 seconds. With the machine running, gradually add the olive oil to make a slightly textured paste. Add the cream and seasoning.

2 Cook the pasta in plenty of boiling salted water for 12–15 minutes, until *al dente*.

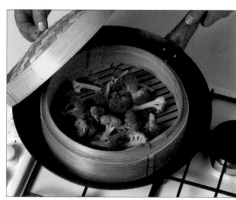

3 Steam the broccoli florets for about 3 minutes, until they are tender but still with a little crunch.

4 Drain the pasta, place in a bowl and mix with the broccoli. Spoon onto individual serving plates and pour the sauce on top.

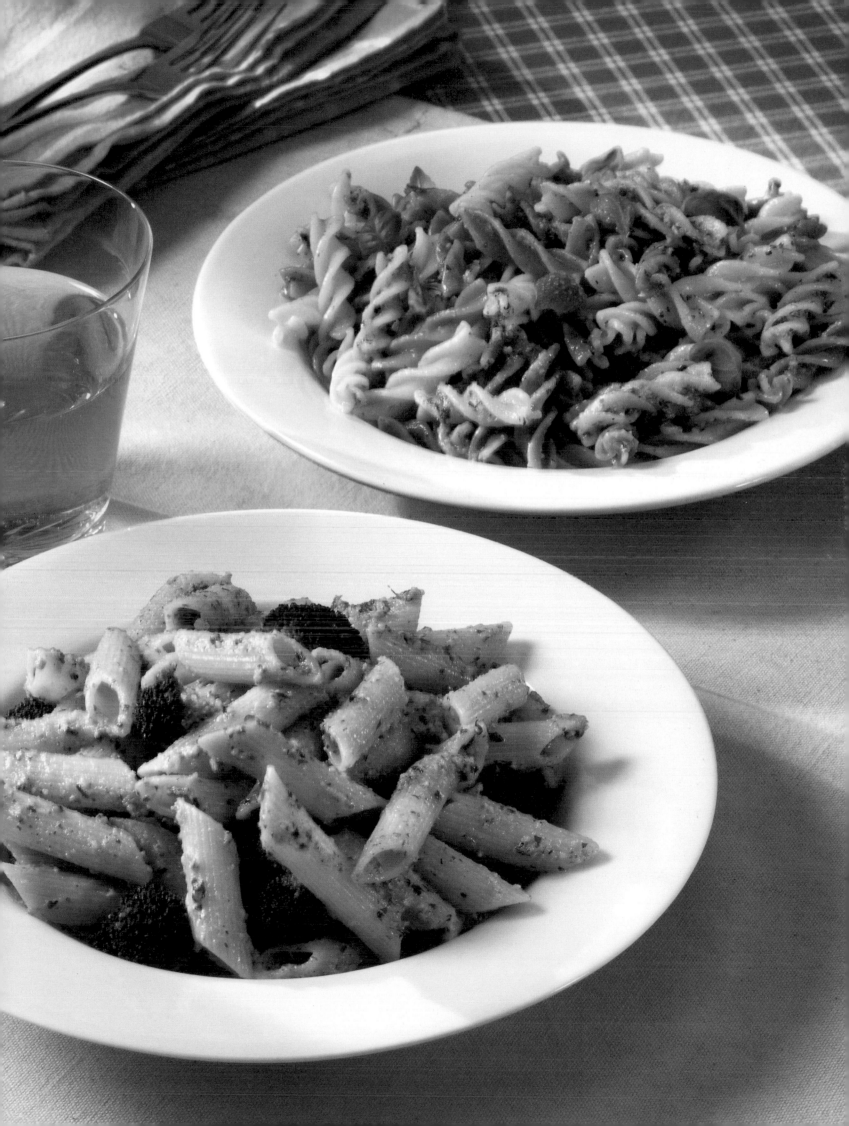

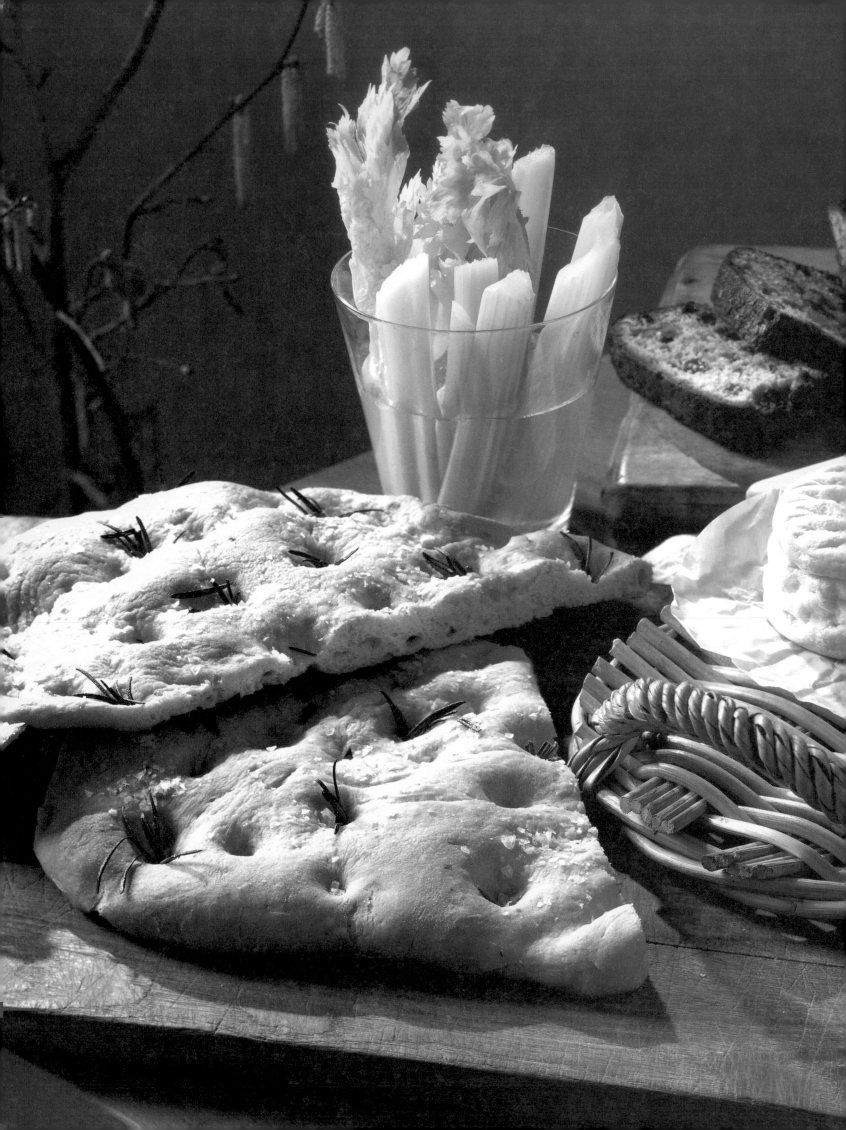

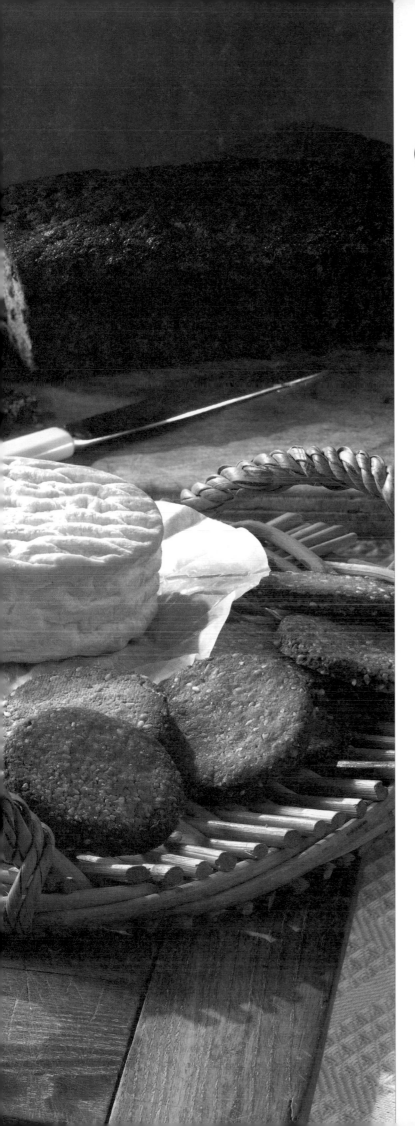

CAKES, BREADS AND COOKIES

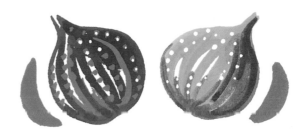

Homemade cakes are much better than store-bought, and prepared with naturally sweet fruits, such as dates and bananas, they are healthier, too, since they require little extra sweetening. Simple breads, such as focaccia, are easy to make at home and worth trying. Cheese and crackers are a classic way of finishing a meal and it is a joy to discover that Sunflower and Almond Sesame Crackers, which are a neutral food, can be combined with any cheese, while Sweet Almond Cookies contain very little sugar and make an ideal partner for ice cream or yogurt.

Walnut Bread (S)

Just the smell of freshly baked bread is appetizing and lingers for hours afterward. This loaf will disappear very quickly and it is wise to make several and put one in the freezer. Serve warm with soups or salad for a light lunch.

INGREDIENTS

Makes 1 loaf
1¼ cups rye flour
1¼ cups white bread flour
1 envelope easy-blend dried yeast
½ teaspoon salt
1 tablespoon butter, softened
1 teaspoon honey
1 cup walnuts, halved
sunflower oil, for greasing

1 Butter a 1-pound loaf pan and sift the flours into a bowl. Stir in the yeast and salt.

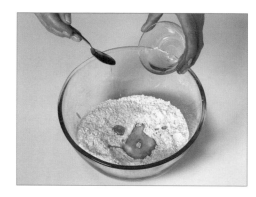

2 Add the butter and honey, then add ⅔ cup warm water and mix into a soft dough.

3 Transfer the dough to a floured surface and knead lightly to make a ball. Place in a lightly oiled bowl and cover the dough with oiled plastic wrap. Set aside to rise in a warm place for about 2 hours.

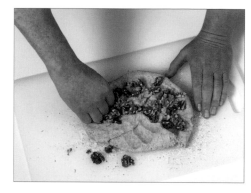

4 Transfer the dough to a floured surface and punch down. Scatter the walnuts over the dough and knead lightly until the walnuts are evenly worked into the dough.

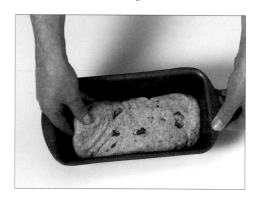

5 Shape the dough into an oblong and place in the pan. Cover with a damp cloth and let rise for about 1 hour, until doubled in size. Preheat the oven to 475°F.

6 Lightly spray the loaf with water, then bake for 15 minutes. Reduce the oven temperature to 400°F and bake for 30 more minutes. To check that the bread is cooked, remove from the pan and tap the bottom; it should sound hollow. If it does not, return the loaf to the oven for another 5 minutes, then test again. Turn out of the pan and let cool completely on a wire rack.

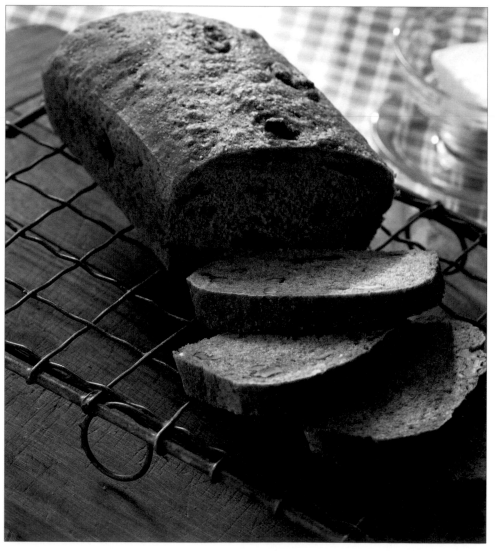

Oat and Raisin Drop Scones (S)

Serve these scones as a snack or as a dessert with real maple syrup or organic honey. If you are feeling indulgent, add a dollop of sour cream or crème fraîche.

INGREDIENTS

Makes about 16
¾ cup self-rising flour
½ teaspoon baking powder
½ cup raisins
¼ cup fine oatmeal
¼ cup superfine sugar
grated rind of 1 orange
2 egg yolks
½ tablespoon unsalted butter, melted
¾ cup light cream or half-and-half
¾ cup water
pinch of salt

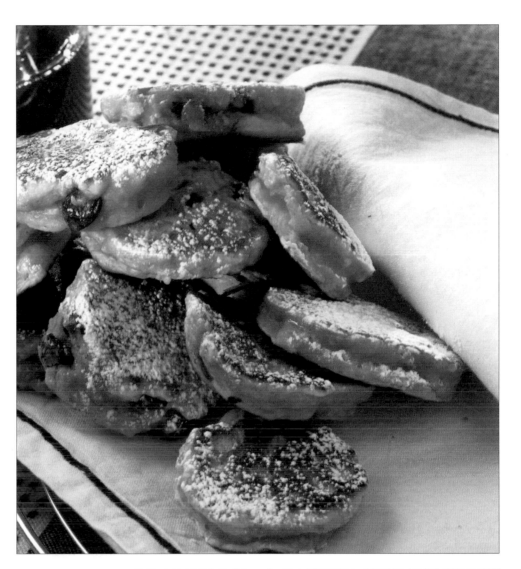

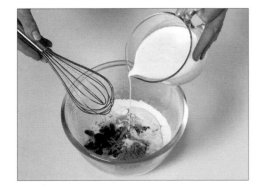

1 Sift together the flour, salt and baking powder.

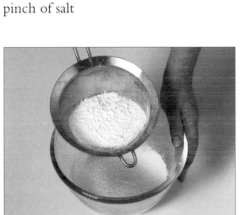

2 Add the raisins, oatmeal, sugar and orange rind. Gradually beat in the egg yolks, butter, cream and water to make a creamy batter.

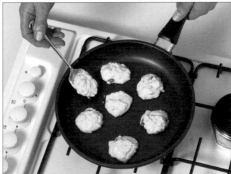

3 Lightly grease and heat a large frying pan or griddle and drop about 2 tablespoons of batter at a time onto the pan or griddle to make six or seven small pancakes.

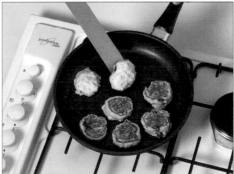

4 Cook over medium heat until bubbles show on the scones' surface, then turn them over and cook for another 2 minutes, until golden.

5 Transfer the scones to a plate and keep warm while cooking the remaining mixture. Serve warm.

Banana Cake (S)

INGREDIENTS

Makes 1 cake

³/₄ cup flour
¹/₂ teaspoon ground cinnamon
1 teaspoon baking powder
²/₃ cup golden raisins
¹/₂ cup roughly chopped walnuts
¹/₂ cup superfine sugar
4 tablespoons (¹/₂ stick) unsalted butter, softened
2 large ripe bananas, peeled and mashed
2 egg yolks
2 tablespoons whiskey (optional)

— VARIATION —

If preferred, use two or three drops of vanilla extract instead of the whiskey.

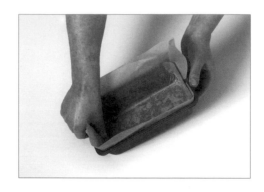

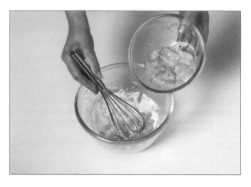

1 Preheat the oven to 375°F. Lightly butter a 1-pound loaf pan and line with waxed paper.

2 Sift the flour, cinnamon and baking powder into a bowl, add the raisins and walnuts and mix well.

3 In another bowl, cream the sugar and butter until light and fluffy, then beat in the bananas, egg yolks and whiskey, if using. Fold in the dry ingredients.

4 Pour the mixture into the prepared loaf pan and cook for 55 minutes or until a skewer inserted into the center comes out clean. Let cool in the pan before turning out.

Date and Honey Bars (S)

Fresh dates, such as Deglet Noor and Medjool, are a good source of natural fiber, yet are kind and gentle on the digestive system. For a slightly different, more toffee flavor, replace the honey with real maple syrup.

INGREDIENTS

Makes 16

1 cup fresh dates, pitted and roughly chopped
3 tablespoons honey
2 tablespoons lemon juice
1¹/₄ cups flour
²/₃ cup water
¹/₄ teaspoon freshly grated nutmeg
1 cup self-rising flour, sifted
2 tablespoons brown sugar
1¹/₄ cups rolled oats
12 tablespoons (1¹/₂ sticks) unsalted butter, melted

1 Preheat the oven to 375°F. Lightly butter the base of a 7-inch square cake pan and line with waxed paper.

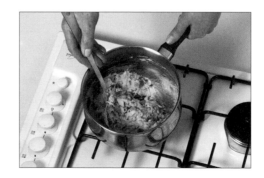

2 Place the dates, honey, lemon juice, flour and water in a heavy pan. Bring slowly to a boil, stirring constantly. Remove from the heat and let cool.

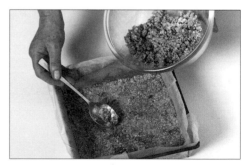

3 Combine the nutmeg, self-rising flour, sugar, oats and melted butter and spread half of the mixture over the base of the cake pan, pressing down well.

4 Spread the date mixture over the top and finish with the remaining oat mixture, pressing evenly all over the surface with the back of a spoon. Bake for about 25 minutes, until golden. Cool in the cake pan for 1 hour, then cut into bars.

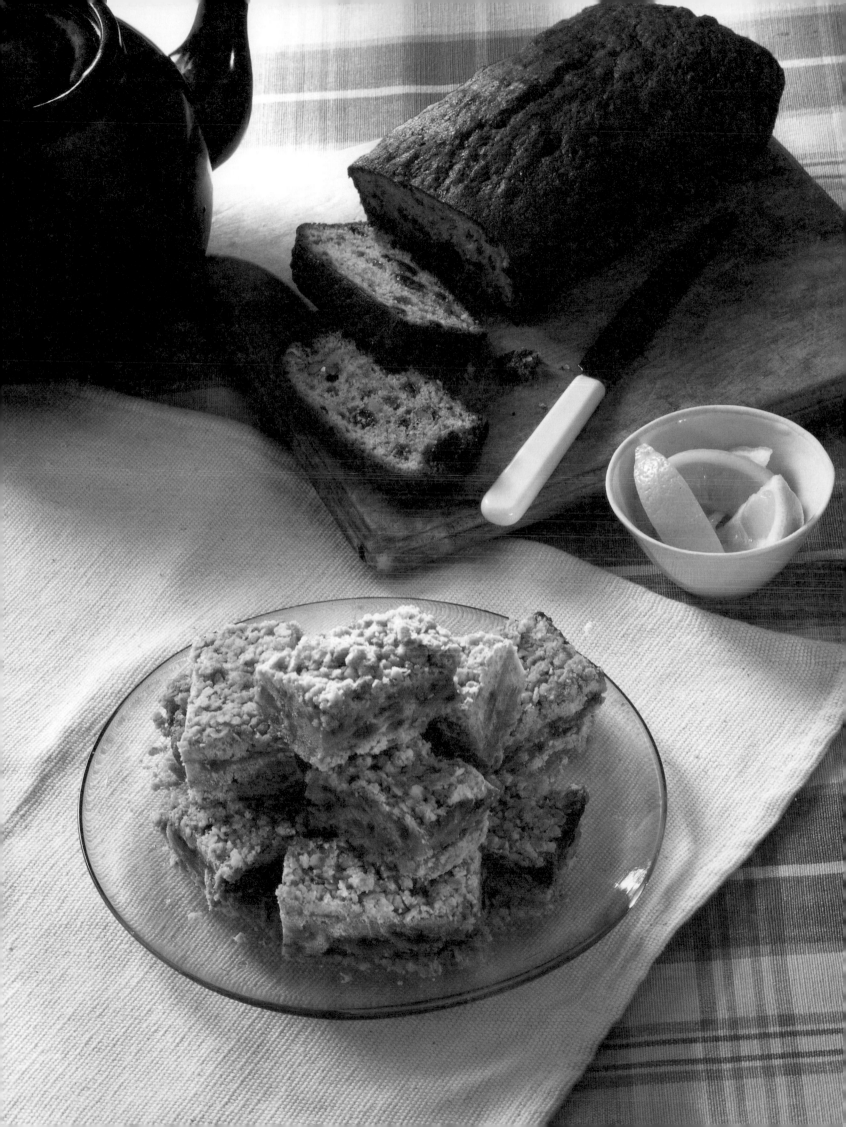

Focaccia (S)

This simple-to-make Italian bread is similar to pizza and needs a really fine extra virgin olive oil to give it its robust taste. Serve it warm with homemade vegetable soup.

INGREDIENTS

Makes 1 loaf

3 cups flour
½ teaspoon fine salt
1 envelope easy-blend dried yeast
¾ cup warm water
3 tablespoons extra virgin olive oil
1 fresh rosemary or sage sprig, coarsely chopped
1 teaspoon coarse salt

VARIATION

As an alternative, instead of rosemary, top the bread with chopped black olives and sliced red onion.

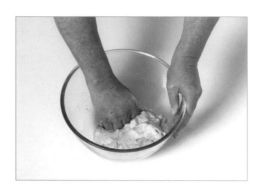

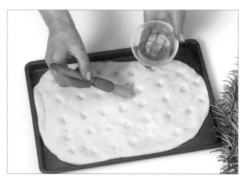

1 Place the flour and fine salt in a bowl, sprinkle in the yeast and mix well. Pour in the warm water and 2 tablespoons of the olive oil and work in with your hands to make a soft dough. Add a little more water if necessary. Transfer the dough to a floured surface and knead well for about 10 minutes, until it is smooth, soft and elastic.

2 Place the dough in a bowl, oiled with a little of the remaining olive oil, cover with plastic wrap and let sit in a warm place for about 1½ hours, until doubled in size.

3 Punch the dough down, knead again for 1 minute, then place on an oiled baking sheet. Pat it out to a thickness of about ¾ inch. Press your fingers into the dough to make indentations all over. Brush the top with the remaining olive oil and sprinkle with the rosemary or sage leaves and coarse salt. Cover with a damp cloth and let rise for about 30 minutes.

4 Meanwhile, preheat the oven to 425°F. When the focaccia has risen, bake for about 25 minutes, until golden brown.

Flat Breads with Fresh Sage (S)

These savory flat breads are easy to make and need no proving or special equipment. They are delicious served with home-made vegetable soups, vegetable purées, hummus or a crisp raw vegetable salad.

INGREDIENTS

Makes 12

2 cups flour
2 cups whole-wheat flour
½ teaspoon salt
20 fresh sage leaves, finely chopped
1⅓ cups water
about 2 teaspoons sunflower oil, for frying

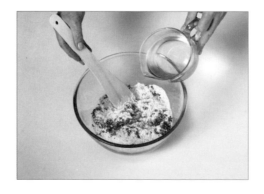

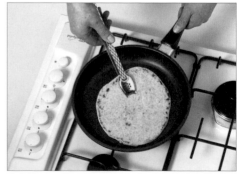

1 Sift the flours and salt together into a large bowl. Add the sage and slowly add the water while mixing to make a soft dough. Knead for 10 minutes on a floured surface, until the dough is smooth and elastic. Cover and let sit for 30 minutes.

2 Divide the dough into 12 balls. Place each one on a floured surface and flatten to make little rounds. Prick each round with a fork. Heat a little oil in a heavy frying pan and fry the breads for 1–2 minutes on each side, until slightly browned and crisp. Serve hot.

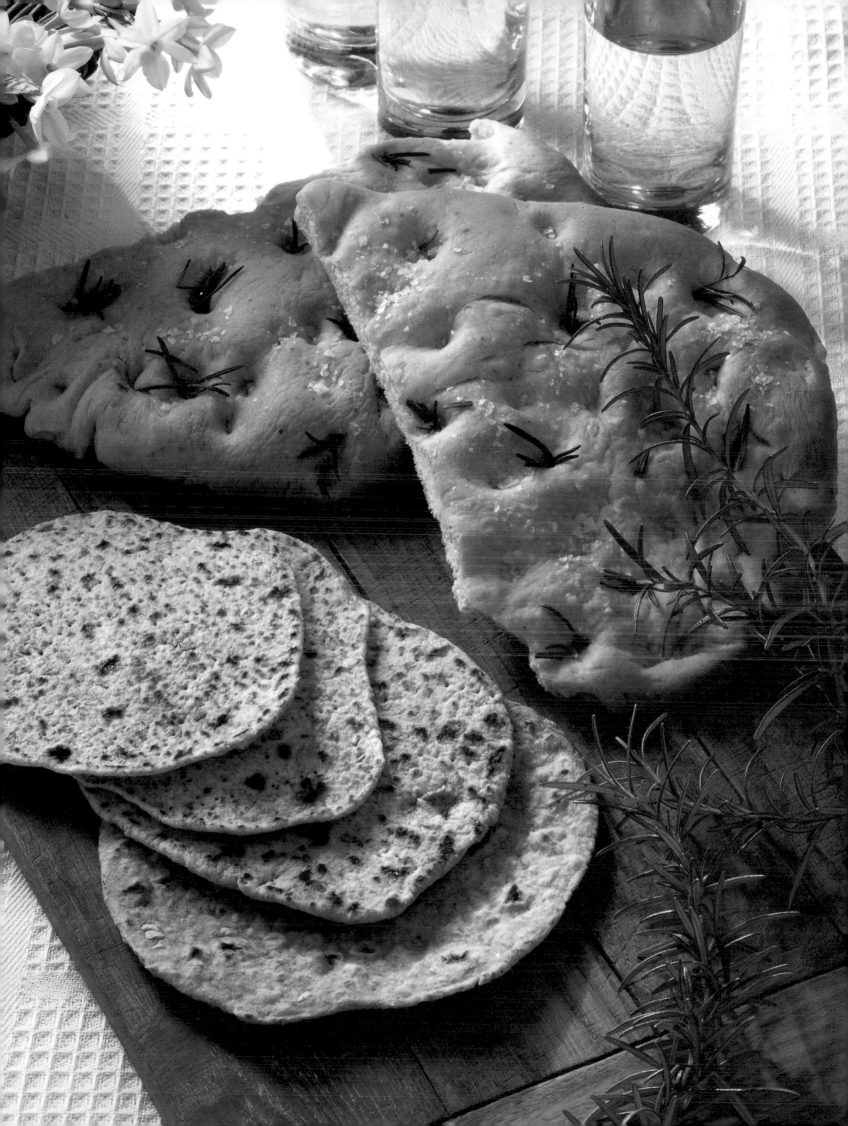

Sweet Almond Cookies (N)

Serve these crisp cookies with ice cream or fruit fool, or more simply with fresh fruit salad, yogurt or a spoonful of thick cream. Make a batch in advance and keep them in an airtight tin.

INGREDIENTS

Makes about 24

2 tablespoons milk
1 egg yolk
2 cups ground almonds, plus extra for rolling out
2 tablespoons superfine sugar
1 teaspoon baking powder
2 tablespoons butter, melted
½ teaspoon vanilla extract

--- VARIATION ---

The egg yolk is not essential but helps to bind the mixture together. If preferred, use an extra 1 tablespoon milk.

1 Preheat the oven to 375°F and combine the milk and egg yolk in a bowl or cup.

2 Mix the ground almonds, sugar and baking powder in a bowl and stir in the butter, vanilla extract and milk-and-egg mixture.

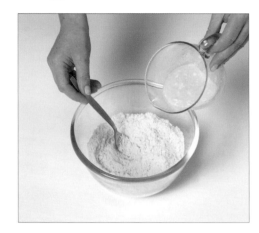

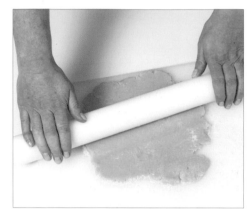

3 Work the mixture with your hands to form a moist dough and then roll out to about ¼ inch thickness on a cool surface lightly dusted with extra ground almonds.

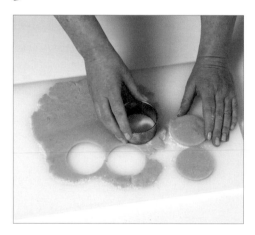

4 Cut the dough into rounds using a 2½-inch cookie cutter.

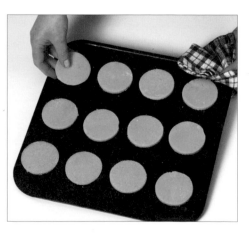

5 Transfer the dough rounds to a non-stick baking sheet and bake for about 10 minutes, until lightly brown. Cool on a wire rack.

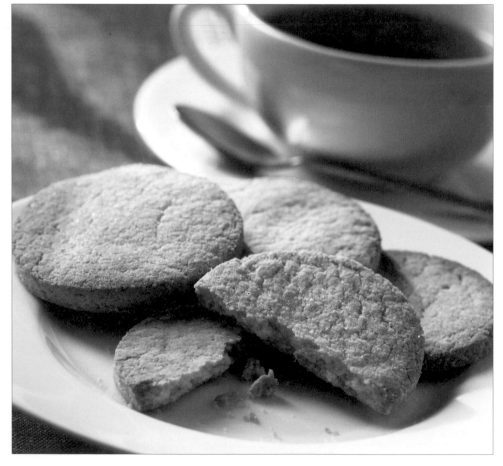

Sunflower and Almond Sesame Crackers (N)

One thing food combiners often yearn for is cheese and crackers at the end of a meal. These neutral crackers can be served either with your favorite cheese or as a base for fish or meat canapés.

INGREDIENTS

Makes about 24

1 cup ground sunflower seeds
³/₄ cup ground almonds
1 teaspoon baking powder
2 tablespoons milk
1 egg yolk
2 tablespoons butter, melted
¹/₄ cup sesame seeds

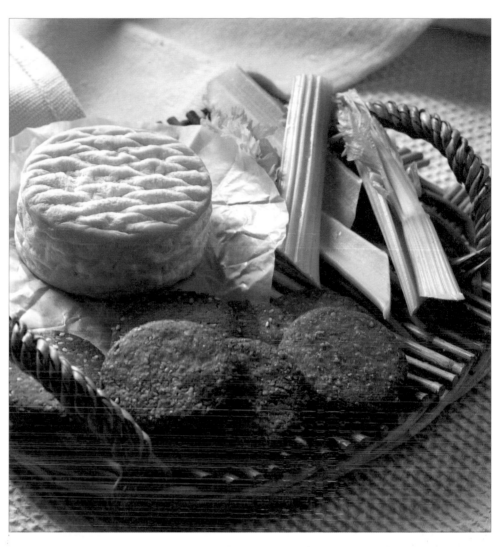

1 Preheat the oven to 375°F. Reserve ¹/₄ cup of the ground sunflower seeds for rolling out, and mix the remaining ground seeds with the ground almonds and baking powder in a bowl.

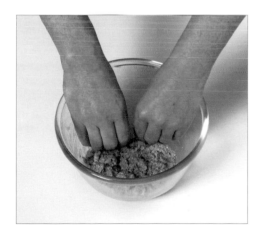

2 Combine the milk and egg yolk and stir into the ground seed and almond mixture with the melted butter, mixing well. Gently work the mixture with your hands to form a moist dough.

--- VARIATION ---

Sprinkle some poppy seeds on top of a few of the crackers before baking.

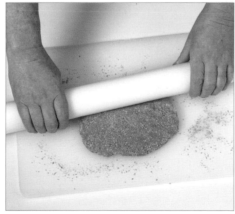

3 Roll out the dough to about ¹/₄ inch thickness on a cool surface, lightly dusted with a little of the reserved ground sunflower seeds, with a little more sprinkled on top to prevent sticking.

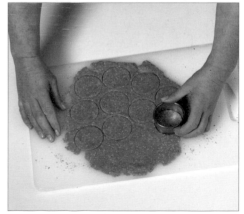

4 Sprinkle the dough with sesame seeds and cut into rounds using a 2-inch cookie cutter. Lift onto a non-stick baking sheet.

5 Bake the crackers for about 10 minutes, until lightly brown. Cool on a wire rack.

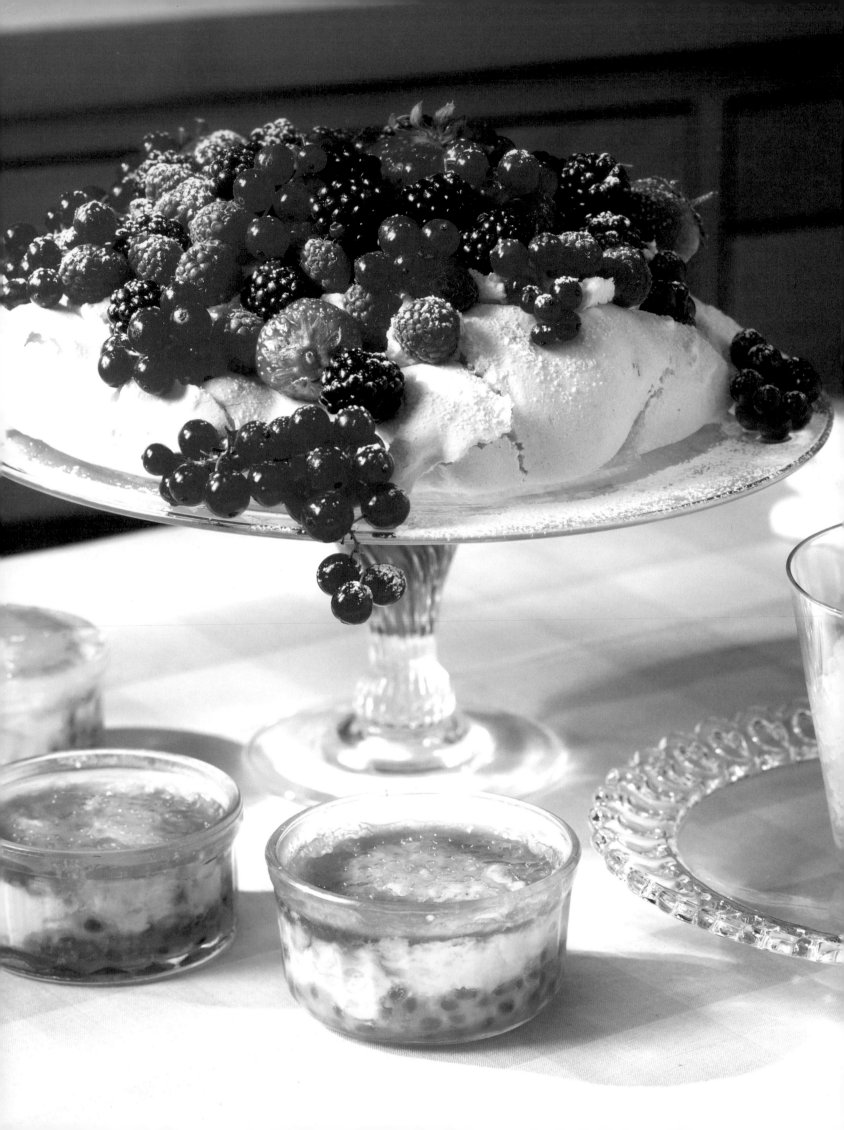

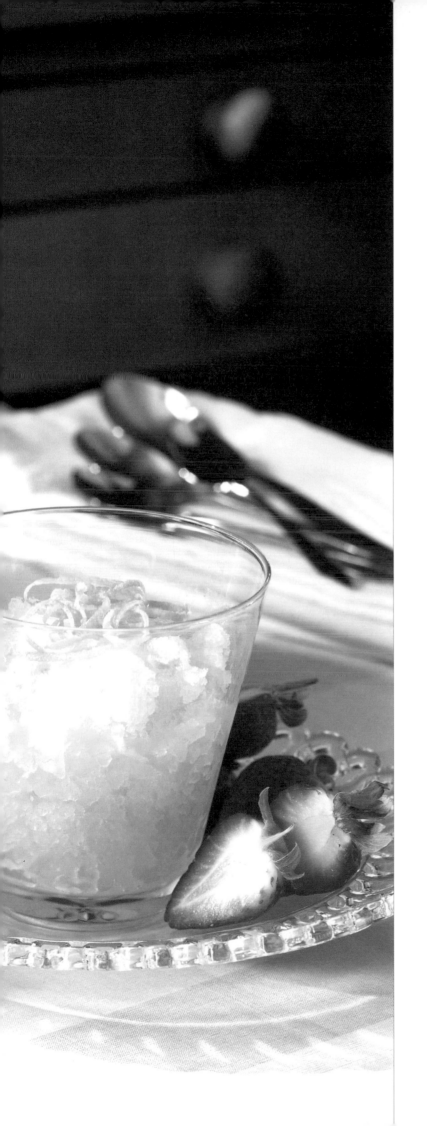

DESSERTS

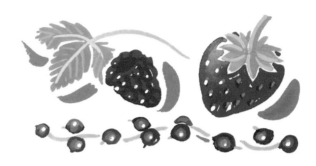

Desserts don't have to be wicked to be wonderful, and a small indulgence does no harm, particularly when it is made from the very best ingredients. When you are planning a menu, remember to match protein desserts with protein main courses and starch desserts with starch main courses. All the recipes are simple to make, and desserts such as Ginger Ice Cream, Passion Fruit Brûlée and Soft Fruit Pavlova are perfect for entertaining, while Pear and Cardamom Sponge will appeal to everyone and could be served at any family celebration.

Sweet Pear and Cardamom Sponge (S)

Choose very sweet dessert pears, such as Comice or Williams, for this delicious dessert. They need to be completely ripe and very juicy. Serve with a dollop of whipped cream or ice cream.

INGREDIENTS

Serves 4
5 pears
10 green cardamom pods
1 cup self-rising flour
1 teaspoon baking powder
generous ½ cup superfine sugar
8 tablespoons (1 stick) butter, softened
3 egg yolks
2–3 tablespoons warm water

1 Preheat the oven to 375°F. Line the base of an 8-inch diameter cake pan with waxed paper, then butter the sides and lightly dust the pan with a little flour.

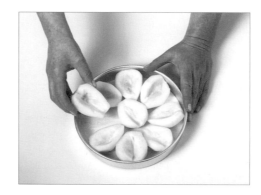

2 Peel the pears, cut them in half and remove the cores. Lay the fruit cut side up in a circle in the bottom of the prepared pan.

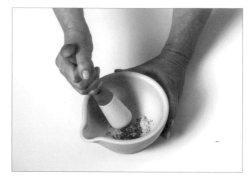

3 Remove the cardamom seeds from the pods and crush the seeds lightly using a mortar and pestle.

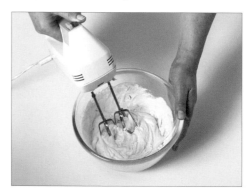

4 Sift together the flour and baking powder. Add the sugar, crushed cardamom seeds, butter, egg yolks and 2 tablespoons of the water. Beat with an electric mixer or hand whisk until creamy. The mixture should fall off a spoon; if it does not, add a little water.

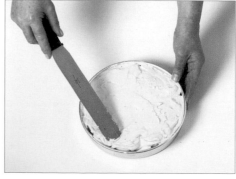

5 Spread the mixture over the pears and level with a knife. Bake for 45–50 minutes, until the cake is firm.

6 Transfer the cake to a wire rack and peel off the waxed paper. Cool before serving.

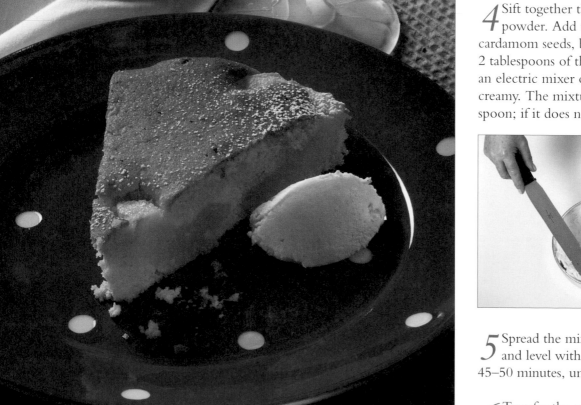

Ginger Ice Cream (N)

This rich and flavorful ice cream goes beautifully with sliced fresh pears and bananas at the end of a starch meal or with gooseberry and apple purée after a protein main course.

INGREDIENTS

Serves 4

1 tablespoon honey
4 egg yolks
2½ cups heavy cream, lightly whipped
4 pieces preserved ginger, chopped into tiny dice

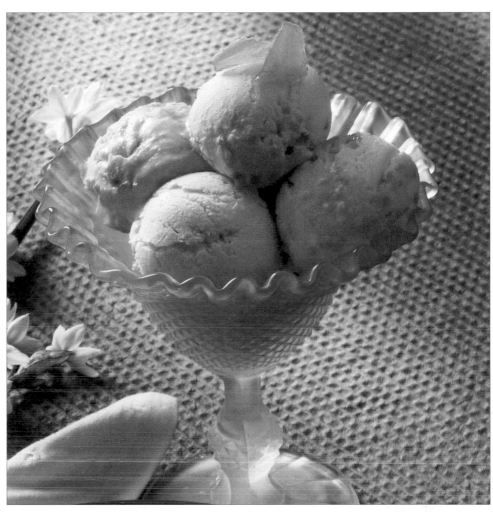

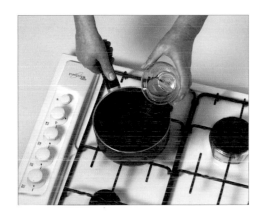

1 Place the honey and ²/₃ cup water in a small saucepan and heat until the honey is completely dissolved. Remove from the heat and let cool.

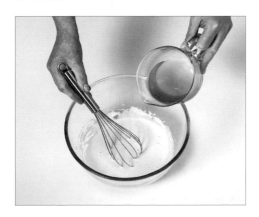

2 Place the egg yolks in a large bowl and whisk gently until pale and frothy. Slowly add the honey syrup and fold in the whipped cream.

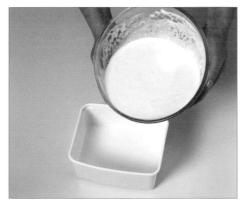

3 Pour the mixture into a plastic freezer container and freeze for about 45 minutes or until the ice cream is freezing at the edges.

COOK'S TIP

Transfer the ice cream from the freezer to the refrigerator 20 minutes before serving.

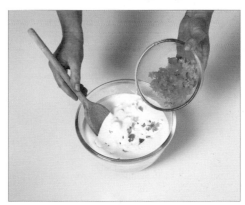

4 Transfer to a bowl and whisk again. Mix in the ginger, reserving a few pieces for decoration. Freeze again for 2–4 hours. Serve the ice cream in scoops, decorated with the reserved ginger.

Passion Fruit Brûlée (P)

Fruit brûlées are usually made with heavy cream, but thick yogurt, which has a rich flavor and is more easily digested, works equally well. The brown sugar required for this recipe is reserved for the crunchy caramelized topping, as the passion fruit pulp is naturally very sweet.

INGREDIENTS

Serves 4
4 passion fruit
1¼ cups plain yogurt
½ cup light brown sugar

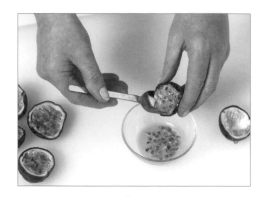

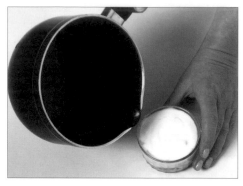

1 Cut the passion fruit in half using a very sharp knife. Use a teaspoon to scoop out all the pulp and seeds and divide equally between four small ovenproof ramekins.

2 Spoon equal amounts of the yogurt on top of the fruit and smooth the surface until it is completely flat and level. Chill for at least 2 hours.

3 Place the sugar in a small saucepan with 1 tablespoon water and heat gently until the sugar has melted and caramelized. Pour it over the yogurt; the caramel will harden within 1 minute. Keep the brûlées in a cool place until ready to serve.

Broiled Nectarines with Amaretto (P)

Amaretto, the sweet almond-flavored liqueur from Italy, adds a touch of luxury to many soft fruits, particularly peaches and nectarines. Enhance the nutty taste by scattering some lightly toasted slivered almonds, still hot from the oven, on top of the crème fraîche just before serving.

INGREDIENTS

Serves 4
6 ripe nectarines
2 tablespoons honey
¼ cup Amaretto
crème fraîche, to serve

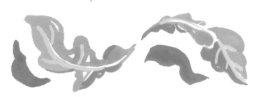

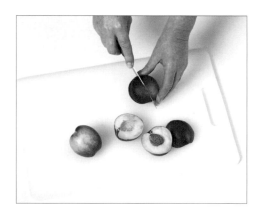

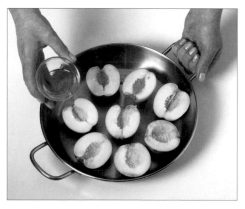

1 Cut the nectarines in half by running a small sharp knife down the side of each fruit from top to bottom, pushing the knife right through to the pit. Gently ease the nectarine apart and remove the pit.

2 Place the nectarines cut side up in an ovenproof dish and drizzle about ½ teaspoon honey and 1 teaspoon Amaretto over each half.

3 Preheat the broiler until very hot and then broil the fruit for a few minutes, until slightly charred. Arrange the nectarine halves on four small serving plates and serve with a little crème fraîche.

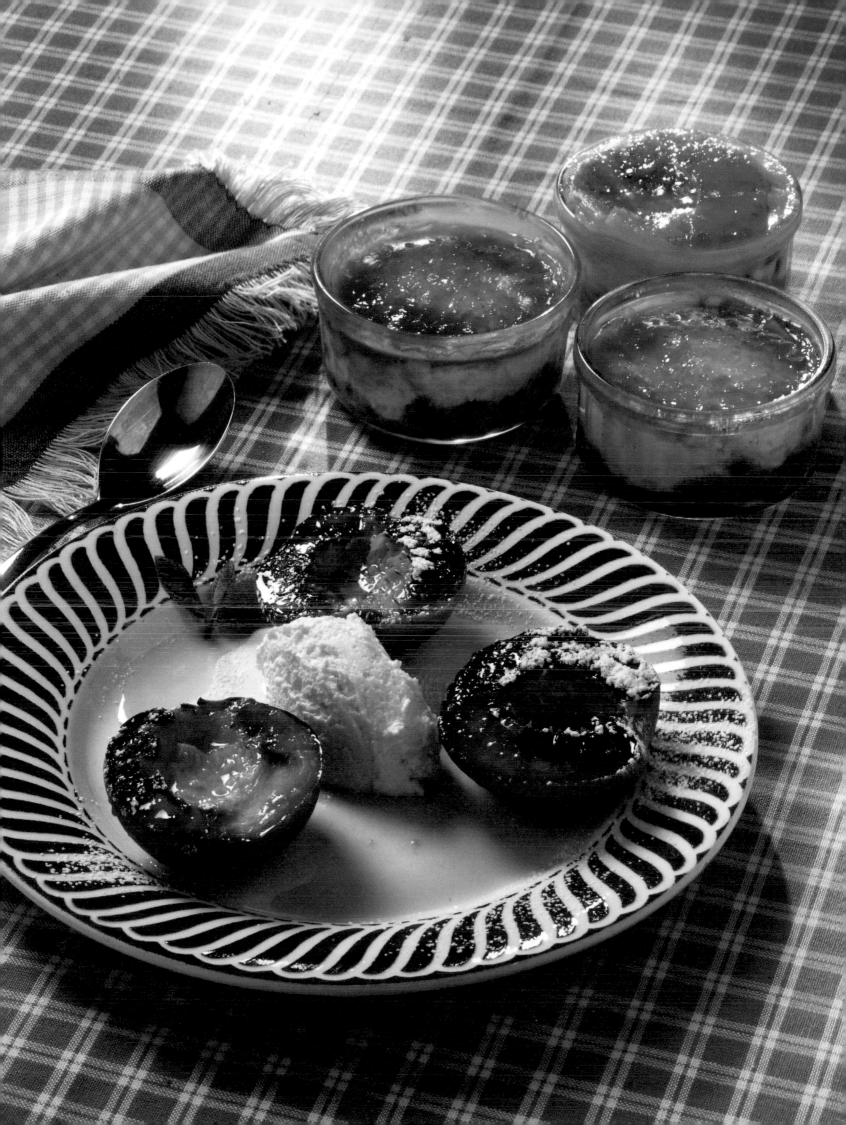

Honey Almond Cream (N)

This dessert is best served after a light main course, as it is very rich and deliciously indulgent. Serve with seasonal soft berries such as blueberries, raspberries or blackberries after a protein meal. Alternatively, serve with slices of very sweet fresh pears or bananas after a starch main course.

INGREDIENTS

Serves 4
1¼ cups cream cheese or mascarpone
½ cup ground almonds
1 egg yolk
1 tablespoon honey
tiny drop vanilla extract
¼ cup heavy cream
fresh fruit, to serve

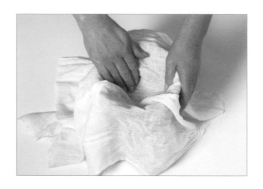

1 Line a 4-inch new or well-scrubbed terra-cotta flowerpot with fine muslin, allowing a generous overhang around the sides.

2 Combine the cheese and ground almonds in a bowl.

VARIATION

A small handful of raisins can be added to the cheese mixture, if desired.

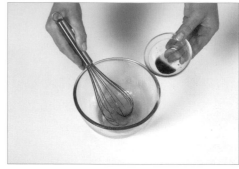

3 Beat the egg yolk and honey in another bowl and add the vanilla extract.

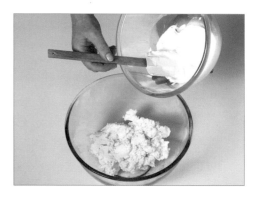

4 Lightly whip the cream, fold it into the cheese mixture and stir carefully until the mixture has the consistency of thick mayonnaise. Add the egg and honey and mix gently.

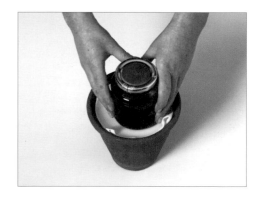

5 Spoon into the flowerpot and fold over the muslin to cover. Place a small weighted plate on the top.

6 Stand the flowerpot in a dish to catch any excess liquid and place in the refrigerator overnight. When ready to serve, carefully turn out onto a plate and serve with the fresh fruit.

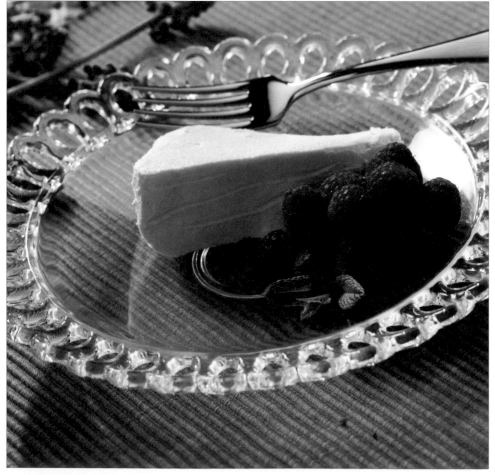

Soft Fruit Pavlova (P)

There is a lot of sugar in meringue, but for special occasions this is the queen of desserts and a practical way of using up egg whites left over after making ice cream or mayonnaise.

INGREDIENTS

Serves 4

4 egg whites
1¼ cups superfine sugar
2 tablespoons red currant jelly
1¼ cups heavy cream, whipped, or
  crème fraîche
1 tablespoon rose water
1 pound mixed berries, such as
  blackberries, blueberries, red
  currants, raspberries or loganberries
2 teaspoons sifted confectioners' sugar
pinch of salt

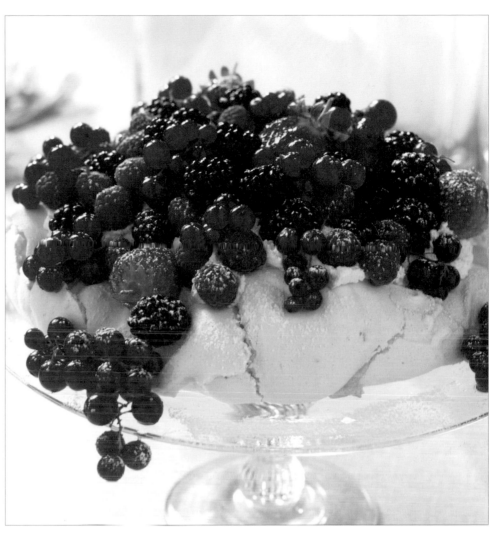

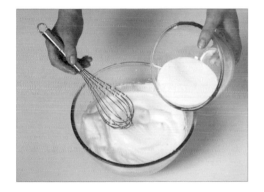

1 Preheat the oven to 275°F. Oil a baking sheet. Whisk the egg whites with a pinch of salt in a spotlessly clean bowl, until they are white and stiff. Slowly add the sugar and keep whisking until the mixture makes stiff, glossy peaks.

COOK'S TIP

Meringues may be made in advance and stored in an airtight container or, better still, kept in the freezer.

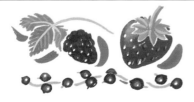

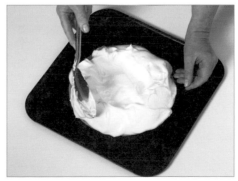

2 Spoon the meringue into a 10-inch round on the baking sheet, making a slight indentation in the center and soft crests around the outside. Bake for 1–1½ hours, until the meringue is firm. Keep checking, as the meringue can easily overcook and turn brown. Transfer the meringue to a large serving plate.

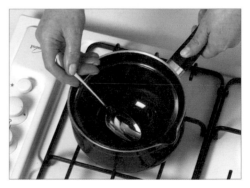

3 Melt the red currant jelly in a small bowl resting in a pan of hot water. Cool slightly, then spread the jelly in the center of the meringue.

4 Gently mix the rose water with the whipped cream and spoon into the center of the meringue. Arrange the berries on top and dust lightly with confectioners' sugar.

Papaya and Green Grapes with Mint Syrup (S)

Papaya is rich in Vitamins A, C and E and also contains calcium, phosphorus and iron. It is very easily digested and has a tonic effect on the stomach, so makes the perfect dessert to follow a richly flavored starch course, such as Filo Baskets with Mediterranean Vegetables.

INGREDIENTS

Serves 4
2 large papaya
1 bunch seedless green grapes
juice of 3 limes
1-inch piece fresh ginger, peeled and
 finely grated
1 tablespoon honey
5 fresh mint leaves, cut into thin strips,
 plus extra whole leaves, to decorate

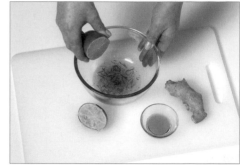

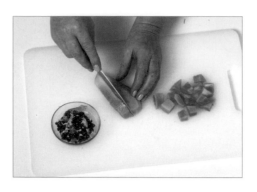

1 Peel the papaya and cut into small cubes, discarding the seeds. Cut the grapes in half.

2 In a bowl, combine the lime juice, ginger, honey and shredded mint leaves.

3 Add the papaya and grapes and toss well. Let sit in a cool place to marinate for 1 hour.

4 Serve in a large dish or individual stemmed glasses, garnished with whole fresh mint leaves.

Orange Granita with Strawberries (P)

Granita is a crunchy sorbet that is simple to make and requires no special equipment. Use very juicy oranges and really ripe strawberries that do not need any additional sweetening.

INGREDIENTS

Serves 4
6 large juicy oranges
12 ounces ripe strawberries
finely pared strips of orange rind,
 to decorate

COOK'S TIP

Granita will keep for up to 3 weeks in the freezer. Sweet pink grapefruits or deep red blood oranges can be used for a different flavor and color. Add a little fresh lemon juice if you prefer a tarter ice.

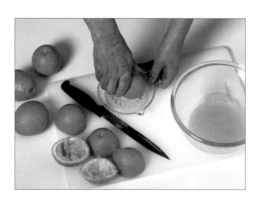

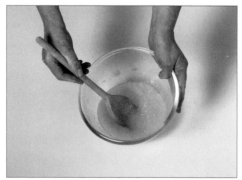

1 Squeeze the juice from the oranges and pour into a shallow freezer-proof bowl.

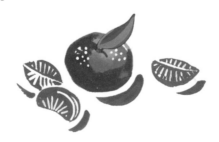

2 Place the bowl in the freezer. Remove after 30 minutes and beat the semi-frozen juice thoroughly with a wooden spoon. Repeat this process at 30-minute intervals over a 4-hour period. This will break the ice crystals down into small particles. Halve the strawberries and arrange them on a serving plate. Scoop the granita into serving glasses, decorate with strips of orange rind and serve immediately with the strawberries.

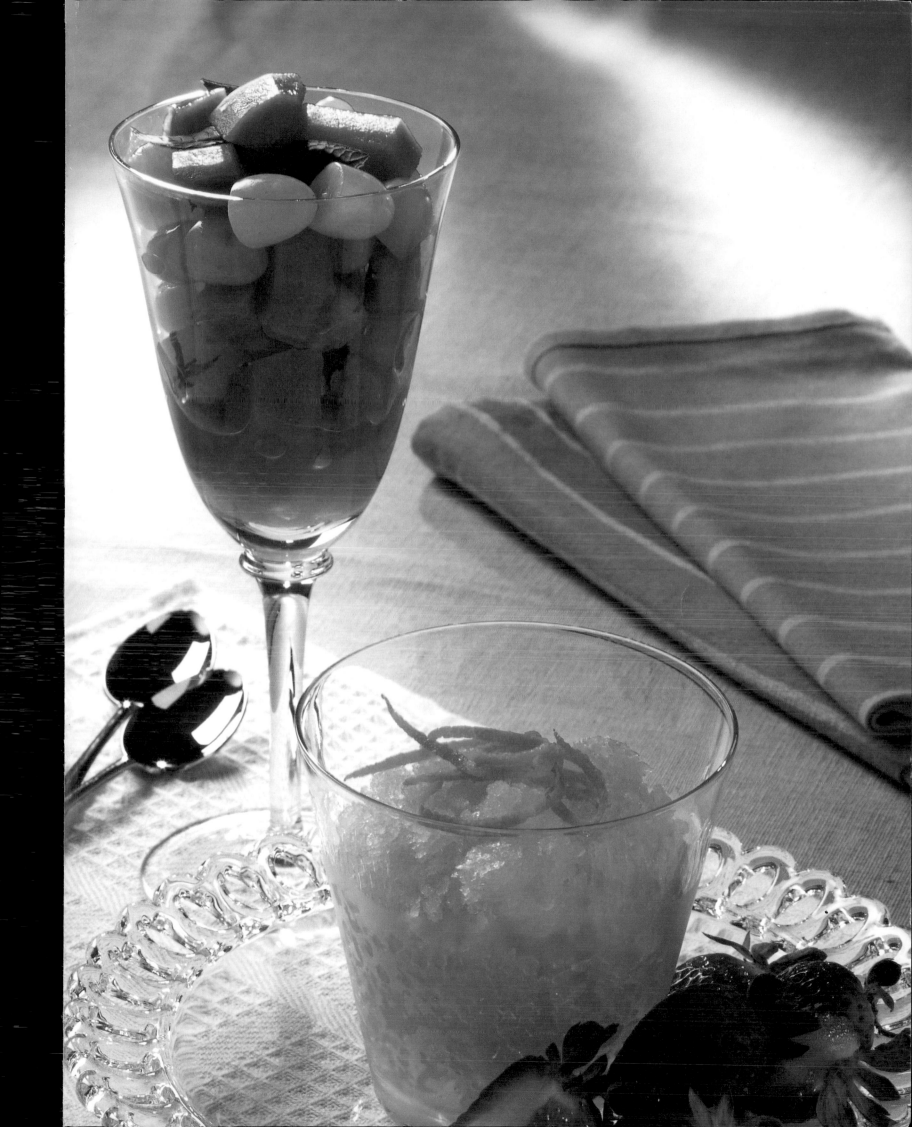

INDEX

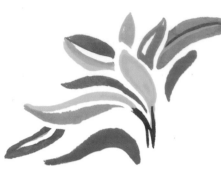

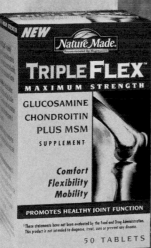
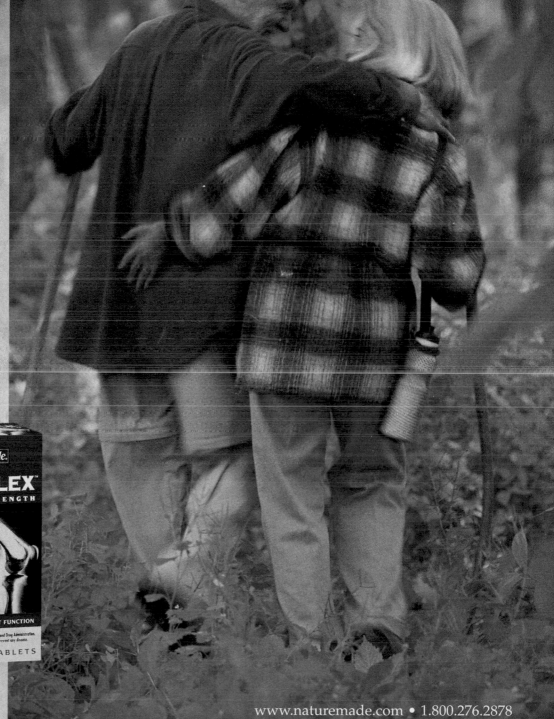

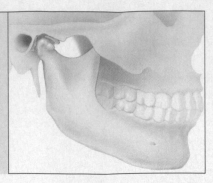

Arthritis

Like any joint, the TMJ is susceptible to arthritis. The forms most likely to affect the TMJ are rheumatoid arthritis (RA), juvenile rheumatoid arthritis (JRA) and osteoarthritis (OA). As many as 10 percent of people with ankylosing spondylitis, a form of arthritis that primarily affects the spine, may have TMJ disorder.

temporal bones to keep the movement smooth and to absorb shocks to the joint from chewing and other movements. Five pairs of muscles, which attach to the lower jaw, support the jaw and allow open-and-close movement.

If you suffer from one of the many medical problems classified as TMJ syndrome or temporomandibular joint disorders (TMD), you probably don't need a simple exercise to find your TMJ. The joint may remind you of its presence constantly with pain, clicking, popping or locking.

Temporomandibular joint disorders are a group of disorders that affects the jaw joint and supporting muscles. Although no one knows how many people have TMD, it is believed to be common and to affect twice as many women as men.

HOW TMD IS DIAGNOSED

In addition to pain, popping and locking of the joint itself, TMD may also be the cause of a number of seemingly unrelated symptoms, including headaches, earaches and dizziness. Because such symptoms can be indicative of a number of problems, diagnosing TMD or its cause isn't always easy.

There are no lab tests for TMD. Your doctor or dentist will most likely make the diagnosis based on a physical examination, review of your dental records and your own description of symptoms. X-rays and other imaging tests may be useful when arthritis of the joint is suspected.

TREATING TMD

For the majority of people, jaw pain is not a sign of a serious problem, and in most cases it is resolved on its own with time.

You can often treat TMD yourself by using hot or cold packs to ease pain, eating soft foods and avoiding chewing gum. Other measures that might help include physical therapy to gently stretch the jaw muscles, nonsteroidal anti-inflammatory drugs (NSAIDs) to ease pain, and relaxation exercises to reduce stress and anxiety that can worsen TMD pain. Some people benefit from occasional injections of cortisone or an analgesic medication directly into the joint.

Because clenching and grinding teeth may cause or worsen TMJ pain, some doctors may prescribe an oral appliance called a bite plate to reduce teeth clenching; however, it should not be worn long term.

If a doctor recommends more drastic treatment, such as extensive dental work or surgical replacement of the jaw joint with a prosthesis, it's important to get a second opinion. Such procedures are rarely required, and in some cases they may cause further problems.

In most situations, a dentist or primary care physician can treat TMD. Depending on the cause and severity of your problem, you may wish to consult a rheumatologist or pain specialist concerning appropriate treatment.

TMD RESEARCH

Unfortunately, researchers and doctors don't completely understand the cause of and best treatments for TMD. Therefore, people in pain may resort to unproven and even damaging treatments when seeking relief.

To better understand TMD and identify future areas of research, the TMJ Association, a patient advocacy group based in Milwaukee, organized a meeting last spring. Scientists working in arthritis, temporomandibular joint pathology, physiology, neuroscience, pain, genetics, endocrinology,

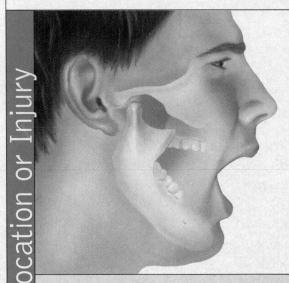

Dislocation or Injury

Jaw pain can occur when the TMJ becomes dislocated, when the disk that cushions the joint is displaced or when the condyles are injured.

immunology and tissue repair, and engineering compared notes on how their knowledge might illuminate the problems of the TMJ and associated tissues.

Anyone wanting to learn more about recent TMD research results or more about TMD in general can visit the TMJ Association's Web site, www.TMJ.org, or write to: The TMJ Association, P.O. Box 26770, Milwaukee, WI 53226-0770.

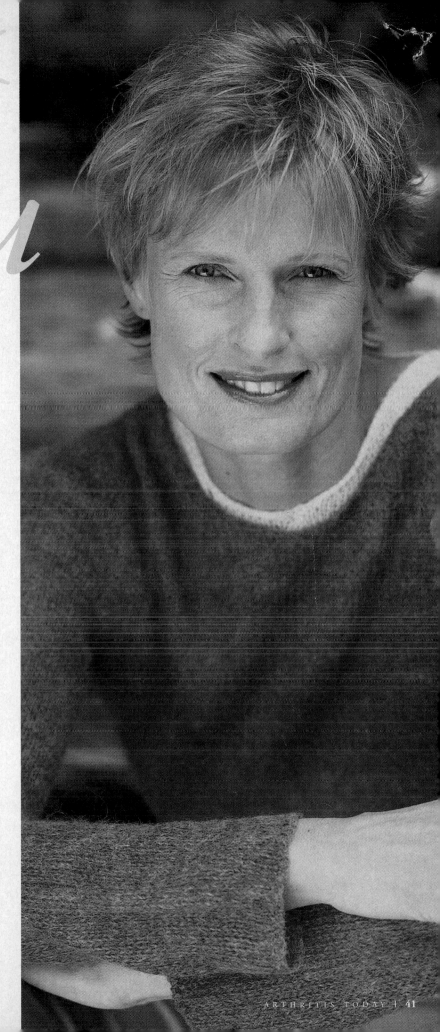

the POWER in *you*

T hink about a time when you tried to do something you thought was difficult or intimidating. Before you knew it, that stressful project, that scary surgery or your toughest exercise routine was over. And while your circumstances didn't change, your can-do attitude allowed you to hurdle the worst and achieve your best.

Thinking positively won't solve all your problems. If it did we'd all be living a life of great health and wealth. It's quite obvious that you can't "positive think" your way to a cure. Before you're tempted to trash your positive thoughts, however, consider this: Your thoughts, attitudes and outlook on life *can* affect how you feel.

As you head down to the final stretch of this year's "You First" Challenge, pay special attention to your outlook on life. Are you constantly telling yourself you can't exercise or beat stress? Instead, use your mind to motivate yourself to try the tough stuff, without sweating and stressing over the small stuff. Tell yourself you can, and you will; tell yourself you can't, and you won't.

Still, it's healthy to recognize your limitations. Don't imagine your success as achieved only if you lose the full 20 pounds. Instead, focus on motivating yourself to workout when you're tempted to hang out.

As you continue on your journey to better wellness, we encourage you to make the most of your mental power. Don't think about all the reasons why you can't do this or that. Instead, make a list of all the things you can do, and allow your thoughts to empower you to overcome your obstacles and change your perspectives about your health. As Norman Vincent Peale, the author of *The Power of Positive Thinking*, put it, "Change your thoughts and you change your world."

– MICHELE TAYLOR

Your Gu

Healthy

What's in your refrigerator? And what about your pantry?

If you shudder to answer, it's high time to purge and replenish. Stocking your refrigerator and pantry wisely is an easy way to ensure that the foods at your fingertips give you healthy options. Deciding what goes into a healthy kitchen determines what goes into your body. Put your kitchen on a diet, so to speak, and you're bound to drop unwanted pounds or maintain your already healthy weight.

The first step toward a healthy kitchen is to start thinking about eating well long before you open your refrigerator or pantry door. So grab a pen and use this guide to compose a winning grocery list. Making healthy choices is easier — and tastier — than you think.

Stock Your Refrigerator the Low-Fat Way

1 Choose fruits and veggies in a wide range of colors to get maximum nutrients, such as fiber, cancer-fighting antioxidants like vitamins A and C, as well as an abundance of phytochemicals. Keep precut veggies and fruits — like celery and carrot sticks, broccoli florets, pepper slices and melon cubes — in the front of your refrigerator so you'll reach for them at snack time.

2 Hydrate your body, control your appetite and get that satisfied full feeling — all at a no-calorie price. Pour yourself a cool, tall glass of water several times each day. New water/fluid recommendations suggest that you drink the equivalent of half of your body weight in ounces. A 150-pound woman, for example, should drink at least 75 ounces of fluid per day. And remember: If you're thirsty, you're already dehydrated, so drink up!

3 For a quick energy boost and a dose of vitamin C, gulp a glass of 100 percent fruit juice like orange or cranberry. But remember, fruit juices lack the dietary

DAVE KIESGEN

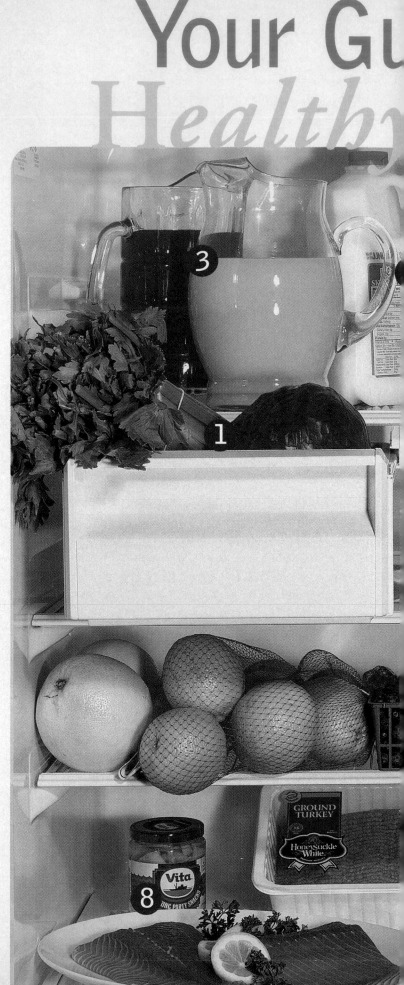

uide to a
Kitchen

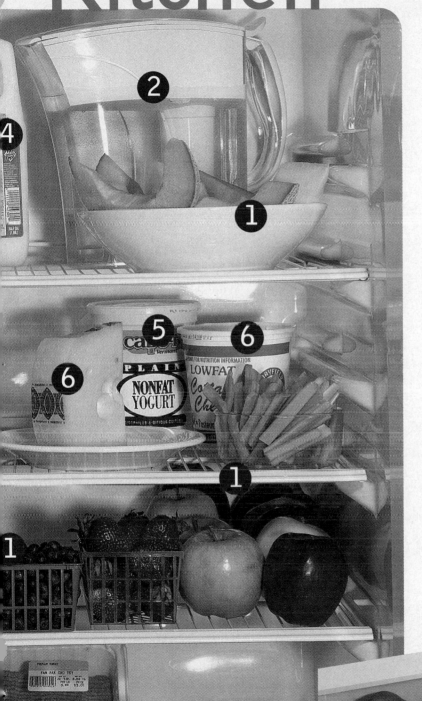

fiber of whole fruit, so don't make them a substitute for the real thing. Also, be cautious of the high number of calories in many juices.

Skim milk provides the same amounts of protein and calcium as whole milk, without the fat. **4**

Did you know that plain, nonfat yogurt is a more concentrated source of calcium than whole-milk yogurt? Try some on a baked potato instead of sour cream, or blend some with fresh or frozen berries to make a fruit smoothie. **5**

Along with calcium and protein, dairy foods like cottage cheese often contain fat. Eat them in moderation and opt for low-fat or nonfat versions. **6**

Boost your protein intake the low-fat way. Eat lean meats like boneless, skinless chicken breasts, ground turkey breast, lean ground beef and reduced-fat sandwich meats, such as turkey, ham or roast beef. To identify lean cuts of beef, look for those labeled "loin" or "round." Meats labeled "select" are usually the leanest. And unless you're cooking a whole chicken, always remove the skin first to reduce fat and cholesterol. **7**

No doubt you've heard that fish rich in omega-3 oil (such as salmon, mackerel, herring and rainbow trout) can relieve arthritis inflammation. But are you eating some at least once a week? Grill a salmon filet for dinner or nibble some bite-size herring pieces (marinated in wine sauce, *not* sour cream) as a healthy snack. **8**

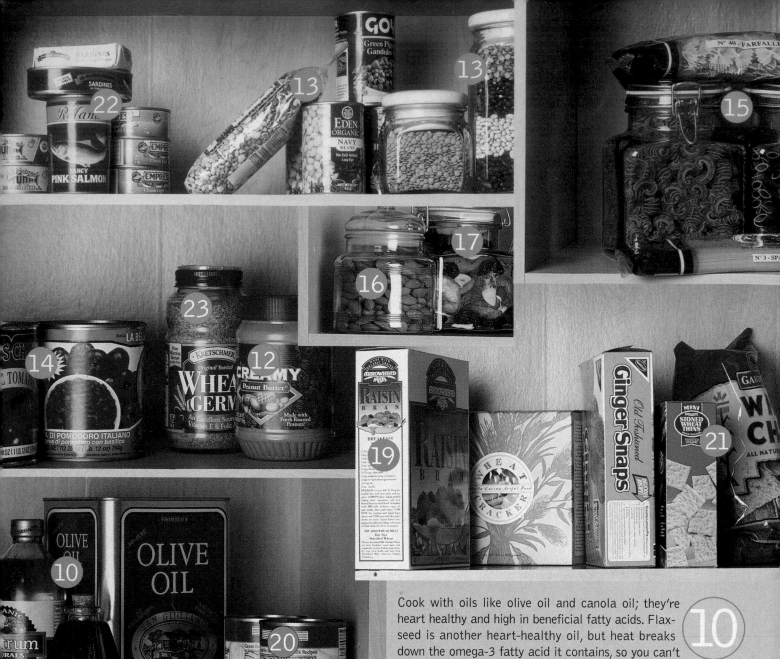

Make Low-Fat Cooking – and Snacking – a Cinch: Pack Your Pantry With These Healthy Staples

9 If the first ingredient in your bread is wheat flour or unbleached wheat flour, the bread is made from refined flour, like white bread. If the first ingredient is 100 percent whole-wheat flour, the bread is primarily whole grain. Opt for the latter, and be sure to eat breads with at least 2 grams of fiber per serving.

10 Cook with oils like olive oil and canola oil; they're heart healthy and high in beneficial fatty acids. Flaxseed is another heart-healthy oil, but heat breaks down the omega-3 fatty acid it contains, so you can't cook with it. Instead, try mixing flaxseed oil with vinegar to make salad dressing.

11 Keep carbohydrate cravings at bay with a bowl of fiber-rich oatmeal at breakfast. (For the most fiber, look for labels that say "old-fashioned, 100 percent natural oatmeal.")

12 Peanut butter is low in saturated fat, high in heart-healthy monounsaturated fat, and it's a great source of protein.

13 Foods with plenty of soluble fiber help reduce cholesterol levels, and beans are among the best sources. If you prefer the convenience of canned beans, choose those without added meat. To reduce the sodium level, rinse canned beans thoroughly with water before cooking or tossing in soup or salad. (Rinsing also decreases the amount of indigestible starches that cause gastrointestinal problems.)

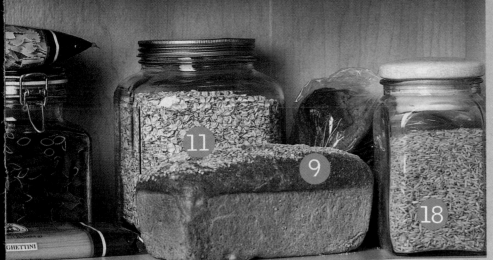

18 Still eating white rice? Face the facts: Even "enriched" white rice is a nutritional weakling. Instead, treat yourself to brown rice – a more flavorful source of fiber and other nutrients.

19 Opt for whole-grain cereals to increase your fiber intake. Try raisin bran instead of corn flakes. Eat cereals with at least 5 grams of fiber per serving to help you get the 20 to 35 grams of fiber you need per day.

14 For very few calories, tomatoes are chock-full of nutrients – not to mention flavor. Chopped or pureed, in salad or sauces, tomatoes are one of the healthiest foods around, providing cancer-fighting antioxidants such as licopene, vitamins A and C, folic acid and potassium. Eat them canned and eat them fresh.

20 For a quick calcium boost, add evaporated skim milk to reduced-fat cream soups.

15 Complex carbohydrates like pasta are a good source of B vitamins, not to mention a quick and easy choice for a low-fat meal. For more fiber, opt for whole-wheat pasta over pasta made with white flour. To balance out a pasta-based meal, add lean protein and veggies.

21 Sure, it's OK to indulge now and then. Choose your snacks wisely, so you can enjoy them more frequently without the added guilt. Eat whole wheat crackers with low-fat cheese. Enjoy a few ginger snap cookies – they're low-fat and cholesterol-free – with a cup of hot tea. And try baked tortilla chips instead of fried, high-calorie chips.

16 While it's true that nuts are high in fat, they mostly contain the good kind of fat (monounsaturated or polyunsaturated). Almonds have less fat than other nuts and they're a great source of protein, vitamin E and calcium. Nosh on a handful as an afternoon snack.

22 Canned tuna, sardines and salmon are natural sources of omega-3 oils, which can ease arthritis inflammation and reduce cholesterol. (In addition, sardines and salmon are terrific sources of calcium.)

17 When fresh fruit isn't handy, opt for dried fruit as a healthy snack. But don't overdo it – dried fruits tend to be high in calories and natural sugars.

23 Sprinkle a couple of tablespoons of wheat germ on cereal, yogurt or a salad to increase your intake of protein, and vitamins B and E. Once you've opened a container of wheat germ, refrigerate it to retain freshness.

THROW IT OUT

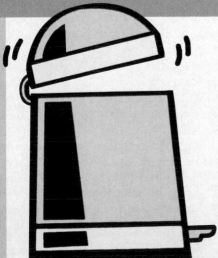

Don't let high-fat, low-nutrition foods sabotage your goals to eat better. If any of these items are lurking in your kitchen, toss 'em today.

- ☾ Full-fat salad dressings and mayonnaise
- ☾ Saturated lards and vegetable oils (coconut, palm and palm kern oils)
- ☾ Whole milk and whole-milk products such as full-fat ice cream and cheese
- ☾ Junk foods like high-fat cookies, cakes, candy and chips
- ☾ High-fat, high-sugar breakfast cereals
- ☾ White bread
- ☾ High-sodium, high-fat (cream-based) canned soups

– BETH BLANEY

"I Am what I Am"

DON'T let that excuse keep you from improving your health habits. **YOU CAN** be yourself and do better. There's no magic involved – just a few tricks.

Most people have heard the saying, "You can't teach an old dog new tricks." Although the statement refers to training man's best friend, many people use it to excuse their own bad habits. "I've lived this long being like this, there's no reason to change now," they might think.

But what if there is a reason? What if, by always being forgetful, you've neglected taking your medication regularly and therefore don't get all the relief you're supposed to? What if, by telling people "I was never athletic," you're not exercising and gaining mobility? Or what if, by being generally pessimistic

ogy professor at the University of California at Berkeley, offers one example.

"You can be a calm, level-headed person, but if you're thrown out of an airplane with no parachute, you'll be in a state of anxiety," he says. "On the other hand, someone characteristically anxious is anxious about everything."

There is much controversy over the theory of traits vs. states. One school of thought suggests traits are simply habits that were established early in life that can be modified. But other experts disagree, stating that everyone possesses some defined,

"We're not talking about changing your personality – we're talking about **changing behavior** that can lead to **better health**."

and negative about your disease, you've alienated people close to you?

To "learn new tricks," it helps to understand who you are inherently vs. how you react and respond to different situations. Experts refer to these concepts as "traits vs. states." Traits are your character traits and your disposition, such as optimistic, aggressive or impulsive. States refers to how you're feeling in a particular situation.

So how do you know the difference between who you are always and who you are today? Jack Block, PhD, a psychol-

innate characteristics that cannot be changed. So, they would say, just as someone is born with blue eyes or brown hair, she also is born shy or athletic.

That might not make you optimistic that you'll ever remember to take your medicine or to exercise, or not complain as much. But don't be discouraged. Even experts who believe in unchangeable traits agree that you can adjust your life for the better.

"Most people aren't trying to change their whole personalities, just a few behaviors identified as important. They want to change so they'll have a better life," says Gene Abel, MD, PhD, medical director of the Behavioral Medicine Institute of Atlanta and a psychiatry professor at two Atlanta medical schools. "We're not talking about changing your